Deborah Williams embodies grace, which, coupled with her innate passion for her craft, allows women of all ages to instantly connect with her. Deborah's approach to beauty is simple, free from the conventional approach that women are flawed and therefore must conform to the societal standards of beauty. She understands that women wear many faces every day, throughout their journey and the many facets of their lives.

Deborah's gift helps women to recognize their own beauty by understanding who they are, who they want to be and who they can be. Deborah helps them to discover their own unique features and how to embrace and celebrate them, thus liberating their confidence.

This is her gift. This is the *grace* factor!

*R. Potrebenko*
National Brand Educator,
*jane iredale*-Beauty With Brilliance Canada


Deborah's colour expertise and proven makeup techniques for the over-50 woman allows every woman to see how makeup can enhance her professional appearance and her beauty.

Deborah's exceptional teaching skills and the *grace* Makeup System shows each client how to duplicate that look in her own home.

I highly recommend *The grace Factor* to every woman.

Bravo! Finally, a makeup book specifically for the woman over 50.

*Diane Craig*
President and Founder,
Corporate Class Inc.

MAKEUP TECHNIQUES
FOR THE WOMAN OVER 50

# the
# grace
## factor

How to look & feel
your best in the
new midlife!

DEBORAH WILLIAMS

*foreword by Jane Iredale*

The Grace Factor: Makeup Techniques for the Woman Over 50

Published by:
Castle Quay Books
Tel: (416) 573-3249
E-mail: info@castlequaybooks.com    www.castlequaybooks.com

Edited by Marina HofmanWillard and Wendy Reis
Creative by David Sharpe
Writen by Carolyn Williams
Hand-drawn illustrations by Carolyn Williams
Cover and interior layout by Burst Impressions
Printed by Marquis Book Printing

Library and Archives Canada Cataloguing in Publication
Williams, Deborah, 1955-, author
    The grace factor : Makeup techniques for the woman over 50 / Deborah Williams.


ISBN 978-1-927355-83-1 (paperback)


    1. Women--Health and hygiene.  2. Beauty, Personal.  3. Aging.
I. Title.


RA778.W554 2016          613'.04244          C2016-905306-7

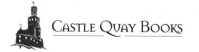

Dedicated to my mother, who was, and is, my inspiration for my grace in life and the reason and inspiration for *grace* Makeup for Midlife.

And to my father, Ronald Williams, who called "Maggie," my mother, the light of his life. He always asked how "gracie" (*grace* Makeup) was doing. Dad would be so proud.

"Learn the rules like a pro,
so you can break them
like an artist."

—*Pablo Picasso*

# Table of Contents

# Acknowledgements

T*he grace Factor* has been a labour of love.

I have so many people to thank and acknowledge: My sister, Carolyn, has spent hours helping me put this book together. My brother-in-law, David, for his expertise, patience and inspiration with the design and branding of *grace* Makeup for Midlife. My business partner, Jim, for all his support and for his endless expertise that has truly taken *grace* Makeup for Midlife to the next level. And my editor, Wendy Reis.

Much thanks to Claude Noel for the exceptional cover photograph and the *grace* signature photograph.

Last but not least, the curious mascots of the *grace* studio: my Cornish Rex and Devon Rex cats, Rupert and Tilly. They are an endless source of amusement and joy.

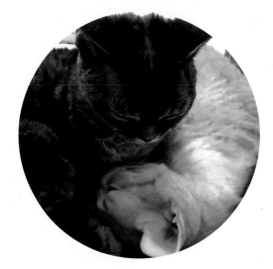

# Foreword

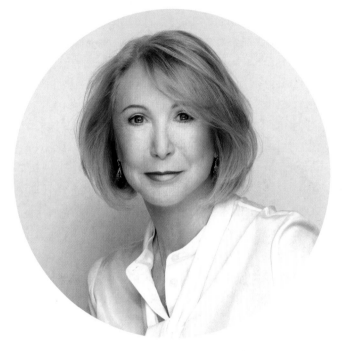

*Jane Iredale, Founder and President, Iredale Mineral Cosmetics, Ltd.*

Makeup isn't trivial! If you don't believe me, listen to Deborah Williams, who says about her new book, filled with so many truths and tips about makeup, that she believes it "will give women permission to be their best." I agree. Makeup is an important part of how we feel about ourselves. In our own studies, we have had women say that when they feel good about the way they look, they do everything better.

Deborah has a simple and effective way of making sure that you optimize your natural beauty. In her words, "Celebrate what you love (about yourself), and what you don't love will fade away." How do you do this? It all has to do with adhering to a few simple makeup guidelines and choosing the right colours.

"Oh, dear," I hear you say. "How do I know what the right colours are for me? There's so much choice!" Don't worry; Deborah has the answer for that, too. She teaches you to find your most flattering colours by learning to recognize your underlying skin tone and how to work with it. No more guesswork. Certainty and confidence will reign.

When I had my "colours done" years ago and found out that I was a spring (warm undertones), it answered many questions for me. Why did so many of my friends look great in black and I looked drab? Why did my teeth look whiter when I wore coral lipstick and yellower when I wore pink? Why did white against my face accentuate the unevenness of my skin? It also helped with shopping. Oh, how it helped. No more combing through racks and racks of clothes hoping that something would catch my eye. I could zero in on the colours that worked best for me—colour swatches in hand. And it always worked.

This colour philosophy is backed up by science. We are all born with a gene that influences the colours throughout our bodies—skin, hair, the irises of our eyes, teeth, even our blood. These genes impart a blue (cool) or a yellow (warm) cast. (Some people think that changing the colour of their hair changes what colours they can wear. It doesn't. Your underlying gene never changes.) Deborah and I believe that working with your underlying colour will enhance your natural beauty; ignoring it can lead to horrible mistakes. For example, purple lipstick on me looks as though I'm headed for the morgue. My warm undertones mean peaches, corals, warm reds.

Some eye shadows can pop the colour of your eyes; others can make whites look yellow and accentuate bags.

Foundation shades can look like your skin, only better, or appear to be masklike. Blush can give you a healthy glow or look as though it were painted on.

Using this as her underlying philosophy, Deborah has written a guide to makeup that includes the best tools for application; how to work with the shape of your face and the shape of your eyes; what products work the best for different skin types; and how to celebrate your age. She is a proponent of not trying to mask the features you don't like but rather accentuating those you do like. I am certain you are going to find answers to questions that have plagued you for years, and you will come away with knowledge that will help you to be the best you can be.

*Jane Iredale*
*Founder and President,*
*Iredale Mineral Cosmetics, Ltd.*

# Chapter 1

# The *grace* Philosophy:
## Beauty from the Inside Out

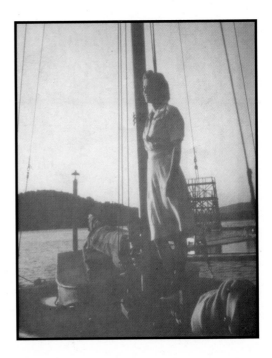

"Don't forget
to fall in love with yourself first."
—*Carrie Bradshaw, Sex and the City*

I have a suit that I call my signature *grace* suit. Forty years old, a lovely soft ivory, it belonged to my mother and, like my mother, is timeless in its elegance. To me the suit epitomizes the classic graciousness that imbues age and aging that is embraced.

Thank you, Mum, for lending me your "graciousness."

This is a book about beauty for women who are aging—us!—in a world that embraces and values youth. I can't make you beautiful in the way you were when you were younger. I can't make you young. But, I can help you appreciate what you have. I can help you be the best you can be.

> "Be yourself. Everyone else is taken."
> *Oscar Wilde*

Such excellent advice, and oh so hard to follow!

Even though it's not always easy to accept ourselves as we are or to be happy with who we see in the mirror—yes, acceptance gets harder as we see the wrinkles and the grey hair—it's something I believe we should and can achieve.

*The grace Factor* is about aging as gracefully as we can. It's learning to be happy with ourselves by actively doing everything we can to look our very best, and it's learning to appreciate our beauty, even when it's a little "wrinkled."

Let's face it: wrinkles and lines, the pull of gravity, losing what we don't want to lose (like hair) and gaining what we don't want to gain (like weight) are part of getting older.

Beauty is not simply about how we look. It's also how we feel. We have to realize that every woman is beautiful even if she doesn't see that beauty.

*The grace Factor* can show you how to uncover and accentuate your individual beauty, and *grace* will strive to help you appreciate and take joy in the world around you.

Benjamin Franklin said there were only two things certain in life: death and taxes. But there is a third certainty, if we're lucky: getting older. We do that one every day.

Every day we're also faced with a choice: to embrace the process or reject it. If you choose to embrace aging, then *grace* is for you.

G generous/gracious/grateful
R radiant/respectful/remarkable
A aware/active/ageless
C courageous/confident/compassionate
E empathetic/elegant/extraordinary

"Beauty is how you feel inside, and it reflects in your eyes. It is not something physical."
*Sophia Loren*

"Youth is happy because
it has the capacity to see beauty.
Anyone who keeps the ability to see beauty
never grows old."
*Franz Kafka*

All right. What does embracing age mean?

It isn't about anti-aging or denying the aging process. (If only it were that simple!) It is accepting getting older, in a way that enhances life and self. It is accepting getting older and appreciating the gift of it, because it is essentially the gift of living. It's about exuberance and fitness, about confidence and peace of mind. And the right makeup!

While we can't stop the aging process, we can make it an amazing and gracious journey. And, with the right shade of lipstick and the right attitude, we can have fun doing it.

The fun part comes after this next colour analysis step.

It's a bit difficult: uncover.

It's the single most important thing you can do.

Uncover your face and really look at yourself in the mirror. Something all of us are loathe to do, I know. Really look at your face and be honest, but be kind. (Kindness to self is very important on this journey.)

Uncovering, looking in the mirror, and liking what you see—hmm. Not always an easy thing.

Each of us has something about our appearance we'd like to change. But if you look at your friends, don't you see something they have that you would like? Those beautiful eyes? That gorgeous hair or skin? That beautiful no-double-chin profile? Yes?

Well, when they look at you they see something that they would love to have.

Still, every one of us has days when it feels as if age is getting the upper hand.

Getting older isn't always easy, and most of us would simply like to stop looking and feeling older.

Impossible?

Well, not entirely.

*The grace Factor* cannot make any of us look younger, but I can help you look your best by teaching you how to enhance your features in a classic, simple way. That will give you confidence, which is one of the most important tools you can develop.

Confidence is key!

It can be your new best friend. It is attractive and sexy and empowering—everything you want to be.

There are techniques and tips about makeup you need to know in order to put together the right look, the one that works for you. Applied incorrectly, makeup can age you, but with the right techniques and tips? Knowing those, you are well on your way to achieving your elegant best.

Colour is another area *grace* can help you with. Not just colour in your makeup but in your wardrobe. The wrong colours will drain your complexion and dull your appearance. The right ones will make you absolutely glow.

So that's how you go about not *looking* older.

As for not *feeling* older?

Again, you cannot go back to being or feeling decades younger than your age. But embracing the aging process is the key to feeling your best.

No one likes to gain weight, to have hair where it shouldn't be and not where it should, to watch spots and wrinkles appear as if from nowhere with every glance in the mirror.

But, you have *choices*.

Regular exercise is a must. It not only retards the aging process; it will make you feel *good*. Feeling good circles back around to confidence and to looking good.

Getting out in the fresh air, communing with nature and appreciating the life around us, feeds the soul. It is essential to both physical and emotional well-being. Take care, of course, that your skin is protected from the damaging rays of the sun. Using a sunscreen is very important, and it should be automatic.

Making wise selections in your diet is another pro-aging choice that will enhance both your appearance and your health. Sometimes, yes, the only answer is chocolate, and there's nothing wrong with that as long as it's not always the answer.

In your life you have to take a holistic approach.

It's not just about the right makeup and wardrobe. It's not just about knowing your body type and choosing the right clothes in the right style in the right colour.

It is about taking care of *you*, inside and out.

So exercise and move every day. Eat properly. Get out into nature. Appreciate your family and your friends.

Celebrate your life.

LET'S BEGIN

*grace* Makeup is a system, for lack of a better word, and the essence of that system lies in a series of discoveries. Makeup is a mystery, and in this book we unravel the mystery by grounding the *grace* system in facts.

If you're going to live in the realm of graceful appearance, there are some realities you will encounter that you *must* adapt to, which will help you live in the disciplines of your grace.

On the physical side, you will be moisturizing, changing eating habits, exercising, limiting your wardrobe and makeup to your colour palette, and taking more time to renew yourself emotionally. These are all realities of growing in age.

As for makeup, knowing your colouring is a crucial element to looking your best. Your hair colour, eye colour and skin tone all compose the mystery of your beauty.

There is a grace to using foundation in the correct undertone and using lipstick or blush in the right colour, all of which will ensure you look your best. Vibrant. Glowing.

Are you an autumn/spring or a winter/summer? Warm or cool? We'll help you learn it all!

# Chapter 2

# The Essentials

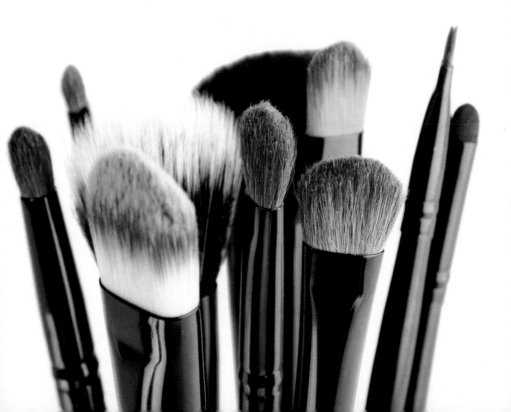

"A girl should be two things:
classy and fabulous."
—*Coco Chanel*

Makeup is easy when you have the right tools! And the right tools are necessary to achieve our best, our classiest and our most fabulous selves. Here is a practical list of the essential makeup tools:

1. Mirror, magnifying if necessary
2. Q-tips for smudging and small cleanups
3. Kleenex for removing excess product and working product into the brush
4. Brushes

And here are the essential makeup products:

1. *Eye Shadows:* Most are powder, although there are crème eye shadow formulations. I personally find that powders work the best. Very often the crèmes "move" and creep into the crease of the eye. The various brands of powder shadows will apply a little differently, and their "stay" ability will vary. An eye shadow primer might help your eye shadow adhere better and stay on longer.
2. *Eyeliner:* There are liquid, cake, pen, pencil, gel, and crème formulations. I find that crèmes are best for an older eye. With liquids, cakes, and liner pens, the application must be extremely accurate because those lines cannot be smudged or smoothed out. They're there to stay. These formulations also tend to look harsh, which makes them aging. An eyeliner pencil is both easier to use and forgiving; the line can be smudged. However, pencil doesn't stay on very well. The crèmes are my personal choice; they can be smudged and are easily applied, they have great staying power, and

they create a flattering softness that liquids and cakes cannot create.

3. *Mascara:* Waterproof, lengthening, thickening, some with fibres in them, curling…there are so many formulations, it can be confusing! Personal preference will dictate a favourite. Colour is the key to using the most flattering mascara. Very black will be harsh on the majority of women and can look especially harsh on a woman with soft colouring. Brown and grey are better choices. Although grey can be difficult to source, for a woman with cool, soft colouring it's worth the search. Brown is best for a woman with a warm undertone. I suggest a touch-up of black to the lashes to add drama at night. (But, if you plan on doing this, don't apply too much mascara before, as it may then clump at the tips.)

4. *Bronzers:* There are powder, liquid, and crème formulations. All three of these are very popular, but I lean towards the powder for myself and for my clients. The bronzer shapes and frames the face. The key to the best application with a powder bronzer lies in using the proper brush. I find that a lot of women just want colour, but a bronzer can shape the face and give you the best of both worlds, as colour and a pro-aging application pop the cheekbones, thus lifting and shaping the face.

5. *Blush:* Blush can be powder, crème or liquid, with powder and crème being the most popular. Both work very well and can be easily applied. Using a crème over a powder could create a "sticky" situation; use crème blusher over a crème foundation, and powder blusher over a powder foundation.

6. *Lipsticks:* Lipstick comes in matte, frost, satin, tint and stain—and then lip glosses and lip glasses, which give the biggest gloss and shine of all. There is also a whole

new line of lipsticks that have all-day stability. So here again, there are so many different formulations, it can be confusing, never mind choosing the right colour! (Although that's something I can help you with). One hint: the more moisture in the lipstick, the less time it will spend on your lips. Some women love the long-staying lipsticks, but others find them too drying. Personally, my long-wear lipstick is one of my favourite cosmetics!

7. *Lip Pencils*: Some are more long-wearing than others, and some, more or less moist. You can either line your lips to define them or fill in the whole lip and use a lip balm over top. This will stay on quite well.

8. *Foundation, Formulations and Coverage*: These come in several forms:

   • *Liquid foundation* is good for normal to dry skin and will give you maximum coverage. If you prefer a more matte look, apply it with a sponge or a brush.

   • *Powder foundation* is convenient for medium to maximum coverage and is always applied with the proper brush.

   • A *tinted moisturizer* is good for normal to dry skin for a sheer natural look. It delivers a healthy glow with minimum coverage. It can be applied with your fingertips or with a sponge.

   • *Mineral makeup* is a "natural" makeup free of preservatives, talc, oil, fragrance and synthetic colouring. It gives full coverage while allowing the skin to breathe. Mineral makeup comes in many formulations, but powder is the most common. The type of application depends on the formulation chosen.

   • *Primer* is often colourless and primes and readies the skin for foundation (similar to prepping a wall for painting). It is applied with a sponge or fingertips.

## BRUSHING UP YOUR BEAUTY

Three factors are essential to efficiency in applying makeup: the makeup itself, the brushes and the application. If one of these factors is inferior, your makeup isn't going to look as fabulous as it could.

Brushes are the most important aspect of actually applying makeup, yet many women ignore brushes as a tool. It's surprising how many women I have seen apply eye shadow with the tiny, useless applicators that come with shadow. Please, throw them away! A Q-tip will serve you better.

Your hands and fingers can certainly be used on your face. As a matter of fact, using a finger to tap the concealer used beneath your eye is perfect, as the warmth of your finger will help melt the concealer into your skin.

However, if your skin tends to be oily, then brushes are a much better option. Nor will your fingers do the fine, precise work brushes are designed to do.

If you find it overwhelming to try to figure out which brush to use for what, this is the section for you! I'm going to demystify the whole process of brushes and brushwork. Here we go.

The different hairs and different shapes of the brushes determine the use of each brush. But, first and foremost, the brush must feel fabulous on your face. If it doesn't, don't buy it or use it.

Brushes can be made of natural hair or synthetic hair.

In the past, synthetic hair brushes were used only with crème products and liquids because synthetic hair didn't grab or pick up powder products. But they've come a long way. Now, my favourite and softest brush is synthetic. It feels like mink and applies foundation powder product perfectly.

There are, however, downsides to synthetic. Because synthetic brushes for powder are relatively new, there's no information on how long they will last. I've had some of my natural hair brushes for fifteen years, and I use them professionally. Synthetic hair also stains more than natural. When you wash natural hair brushes, the powder colour comes out, but this isn't the case with the synthetic hair.

There are many types of natural hair brushes to choose from: goat, pony, sable, squirrel and badger are among the most common. And among these different hair types are subcategories. For example, sable comes from mink, and there are three types of sable—Kolinsky (the best), red sable and sable.

Different hairs are also shaped differently. A brush made of pony and goat hair will not come to a point. These are flat at the tip, and they're wonderful for applying blush and powder. Sable and squirrel hair brushes, on the other hand, are conical in shape, coming to a point, which makes them fabulous for applying eye shadow.

There are prepackaged sets of brushes that seem to have a few that even I, as a makeup artist, can't figure out what to do with! Why buy a set of ten or more brushes if you can't use all of them? Makeup brushes are an investment and can last five years or longer, depending on the type of hair used and the care they receive.

On a daily basis, when you use any brush in a powder, you should brush it across a tissue to get rid of excess powder. Flip the brush back and forth a number of times or gently wipe the brush on a tissue. For brushes used in a crème product, wipe the excess crème on a tissue.

Personal makeup brushes need to be washed, not every day but only if they have an odour or have beads of makeup on them. If, however, you have oily skin, the brushes may get dirtier and may develop a greasiness that will interfere with the makeup application. They might also develop bacteria, so washing is in order.

To wash your brushes, use soap gentle enough for woolens and delicate clothes.

1. Dissolve the soap in warm water.
2. Gently swish the brush around up to the ferrule. Use your fingers in the hairs to stroke the hair from root to tip.
3. Rinse brush thoroughly in running water till the water runs clean.
4. Brush the excess water out of the brush on a soft towel.
5. Stroke the brush to reshape or use a small comb through the hair from root to tip.
6. If the brush does not reshape, use a very small amount of non-alcoholic hairspray. Spray it in your hand, and very gently stroke the brush from root to tip.
7. Lay the brushes down on a towel to dry flat. If the brush heads are over the edge of the counter, the air will dry them more quickly and they won't flatten out on one side. You can stand them up as long as there is no excess water, as you do not want water to run into the ferrule.

If you use alcohol on your brushes they will wear out faster, as alcohol can strip the natural oil in the hair. (Professional makeup artists use alcohol very often because it dries quickly, and the brush can be used on another person within five to seven minutes.) There are specialized brush cleaners, but I have found them to be too strong, and they can stain the brushes. Once in a while, if you need to clean the brushes right away, 99 percent alcohol can be used, but make sure not to get the ferrule in the alcohol or it will loosen the glue and could release the brush.

In chapter 9, I further explain how to load the brushes and how to use them correctly.

## HOW TO USE YOUR MAKEUP BRUSHES

First load your brush with product. Gently sweep the brush across the product in the direction of the bristles. A quality brush will grab the product; it's not necessary to use a lot of pressure when loading the brush.

For your foundation powder, once the flat-top brush is loaded, take a look at it to make sure that you are using the correct pressure to grab the powder foundation. Wherever you place the brush first is where you will deposit the greatest amount of the product. On the face we very often have more redness throughout our cheek area, so once the brush is loaded with product, place the brush in the cheek area first and move towards the jawline and into the nose area. By then you will need to reload your brush. Hold this brush with your thumb and index finger, resting the brush between these two digits. This will give you the greatest control.

For the brushes with longer handles, hold the brush as you would a pencil. Use short back and forth movements in a windshield wiper fashion. Gently press the brush into the face, "tapping" (stippling) to apply the foundation powder.

By using the brushes this way you will create the cleanest application.

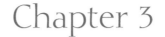

Chapter 3

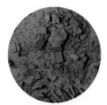

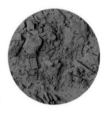

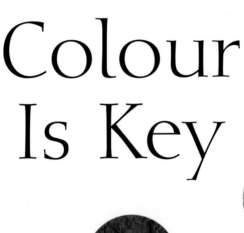

# Colour
# Is Key

"The best colour in the world
is the one that looks best
on you."
—*Coco Chanel*

olour is one of nature's greatest gifts. Diversity, creativity, imagination—they are all sparked through the gift of colour. Colour dazzles and enthralls and delights the eye. And colour is key to bringing out the best and most beautiful you.

I'm here to help you figure out your skin tone and which makeup colours will suit you.

When I talk about colour and makeup, I'm referring to *skin undertone*. Are you warm (yellow undertones) or cool (pink undertones)? Warm and cool determine colour choice, from foundation to lipstick and everything in between.

The categorizing of cool and warm colours to improve appearance by choosing the colours that enhance a woman's skin tone, eye colour and hair colour started in the 1970 book titled *Colour Me Beautiful*, written by Carole Jackson. I remember my mother getting her colours done and buying this book.

Carole Jackson divided colour into seasons: winter, summer, spring, and autumn, with winter and summer being the cool seasons, spring and autumn being the warm seasons.

If you're not sure whether you are warm or cool, here is a way that will help. This is something I do with my clients and something you can do at home.

First, you will need a piece of silver reflective material and a piece of gold. The material must be reflective to determine your colouring.

Sit in front of a mirror and drape the gold and silver materials across your chest and up to your neck and across your shoulders, gold on top of silver (or the other way around, of course!).

Does the gold that reflects on your face even out your skin tone?

Remove the gold to reveal the silver, and look at your skin tone again. Does the silver even out your skin tone better than the gold?

Do this again, this time picking out one spot on your face—try the "bags" under your eye. (We all have those!) Does the gold make the bags look better or worse? Does the silver?

You can do this several times, concentrating on several different areas of your face, until you are sure which colour works better to even out your skin tone and give you a healthy overall glow.

If the gold is better, you are warm, a spring or an autumn season.

If the silver is better, you are cool, a winter or a summer season.

Once you know your skin undertone, you will never make a bad makeup purchase! And, if you know what colours work with your skin tone, the rest is easy.

Now we can continue.

## COOL WINTER AND SUMMER SEASONS

Winter colours are the jewel tones: emerald green, ruby red, sapphire blue. It's the cool season that successfully wears white and black.

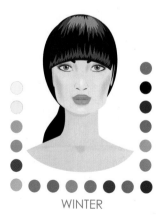

WINTER

You are in the winter category if you have dark brown or black hair with a cool blue or a taupe undertone.

Winter eyes are dark brown or a cool dark blue or black or grey; there are no gold flecks in the winter eye. If you have gold flecks or any gold colour in your eye, you will be a warm autumn or spring.

The winter complexion is milky with a pink undertone. A darker brown or black complexion will often have a blue undertone.

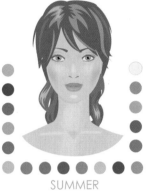

SUMMER

You are in the summer category if you have taupe blonde or taupe brown hair.

Summer colours are the pearly and smoky colours, like grey.

Summer eyes are soft clear blue or green.

The summer complexion is milky or porcelain.

If you are summer or winter, your hair will go white or grey, and it is usually a very striking colour.

## WARM SPRING AND AUTUMN SEASONS

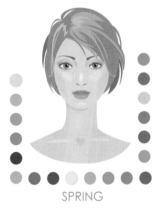

SPRING

Spring colours are all tints—that is, any colour mixed with white—light and bright colours.

Autumn colours are the earth tones, the orange-browns.

You are in the spring category if you have blonde or brown hair with golden undertones.

Spring eyes are green, blue or soft brown. There is usually a sparkle to the eye that gives the appearance of spokes or rays around the iris. Gold flecks are common with the green and hazel eyes.

The spring complexion is warm with a yellow undertone.

You are in the autumn category if you have light golden brown or red to deep auburn hair.

Autumn eyes are green, medium-blue, turquoise, or warm brown, with golden flecks.

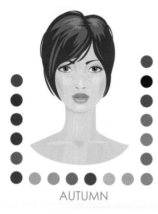

AUTUMN

The autumn complexion is warm with a yellow undertone, and freckles are common in someone with red hair.

Today, the theory of seasonal colours recognizes that some women flow from one season to another. For example, a winter can flow into a deep autumn, which means that women who do this can wear the deep, rich autumn colours as well as the jewel tones of winter.

For the purposes of makeup, I will refer to someone having a warm or a cool undertone.

The concern is to match the makeup foundation with the intensity (the depth of colour of skin) and the undertone of warm or cool, yellow or pink, of the skin. The warm or cool undertone will also be considered when choosing all the other makeup products, from eye shadow and liner to blush and lipstick.

If you are warm and want to use natural earth tones, you would go into the natural warm browns. If you are cool, you would turn to the natural cool browns, which usually have grey in them.

MY *jane iredale* CHOICE

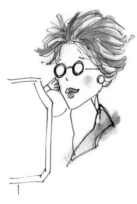

There was no doubt when I was born that I was a redhead. As my mother told me, there were three babies: blonde, brunette and redhead. I was a true carrottop. Bright copper-red hair and blue-turquoise sparkly eyes. My sister was more of a strawberry-blonde redhead with hazel eyes and softer colouring than me. My niece has deep chestnut red hair, dark chocolate-brown eyes and black eyelashes and brows.

The majority of redheads have a warm yellow or peachy undertone, but they can fall into a deep autumn, such as my niece, or softer "autumn or spring" colouring, as for me or my sister. The intensity and depth of warmth will be different from woman to woman, but the warm yellow undertone will differentiate from the cool pink undertone of the woman who is a winter or summer.

The *jane iredale* line of products is divided into warm, cool and neutral undertones, categories that complement the different colouring each woman has.

Throughout each chapter I will give you my personal *jane iredale* choices.

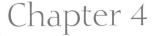

# Chapter 4

# Foundation, Primer, Concealer

"Beauty without grace
is the hook without bait."
—*Ralph Waldo Emerson*

oundation is the cornerstone of the *grace* Makeup System.

Clean, beautiful makeup starts with a clear, even palette. Whether you are 20 or 60, your skin is the largest organ of your body. The older I get, the more aware and concerned I am about what I put on my skin and what I put into my body. This is the *grace* woman mentality.

That is why foundation is the cornerstone of the *grace* Makeup System. It was really important when I started *grace* Makeup that I chose a line of makeup that not only performed at the highest level but was also beneficial to the health of my skin and the health of my clients' skin. The *jane iredale* line of makeup was the answer for me and my clients.

In this chapter, I have included a description of all types of foundations and formulations. It's important to know that most of the different formulations can be made in a mineral format.

## FOUNDATION

Foundation is a skin-coloured cosmetic applied to the face to give the complexion an even, uniform colour and to cover flaws. The first commercially available foundation was Max Factor's Pan-Cake, such a huge success that it is still available today, more than 70 years later.

I think that evening out our skin tone is one of the most de-aging or pro-aging things we can do. As we age, our skin becomes finer. Thinner. Little imperfections show through. Creating an even palette shows off our beautiful eyes and lips and cheeks.

I encounter many women who don't like the feel of makeup on their skin. They feel it clogs the pores. They feel like they're wearing a mask. However, there are so many different formulations, colours and textures that everyone can find one that feels good on her skin. Also, many foundations have sun protection and active ingredients for skin maintenance, which are a bonus.

There are a number of factors to take into consideration when choosing a makeup foundation. Colour is key. The majority of cosmetic companies make warm, cool and neutral colour tones.

Another important factor to consider is coverage, the opacity of the foundation, that is, the degree to which the makeup covers your skin and conceals imperfections. There are many formulations, from sheer to full coverage. Sheer is the most transparent. Very often, tinted moisturizers give a sheer coverage. Medium will give more coverage. Full is more heavily pigmented and will give maximum coverage.

## FOUNDATION FORMULATIONS

Liquids have, in the past, been the most common. They are usually oil based.

Powder-based foundations emerged in the past fifteen years. They give a light to full coverage, and many can be used wet or dry.

Silicone-based foundations have been introduced in the last five years. They're a blend of water and silicone and tend to slide onto the face and spread well.

Mineral-based foundation first came out as a powder, but now it can be found in every formulation, from liquid to powder to crème. Mineral makeup can go from a sheer to a full coverage.

Stick foundations are very common and have been around for a long time. They generally provide full coverage.

There is also makeup mousse and airbrushing.

This is a just a sample of what is available today. You can get any formulation and coverage you desire. So, there is a foundation for everyone!

## HOW TO CHOOSE YOUR FOUNDATION

You need a foundation, and you don't know where to start. If you haven't worn foundation in years, the number of choices can seem overwhelming. There are so many! But, all those choices mean that there is something out there you will love. You just have to find it.

How the foundation feels on your skin and the ease of application will most likely determine which one is for you. So, you have to try them on. Don't, however, try to buy foundation "off the rack" without trying it on. The colour will not be the same out of the bottle as on your skin.

With trying foundation on your skin as the first step in your makeup journey, get a professional recommendation. Go to a qualified person and place to get both the choice and the recommendation.

Make sure you know your colouring or that the person you've chosen to help you is knowledgeable. Go with a clean face so you can try foundation on your cheek. If the chosen colour is slightly off, go one shade up or one shade down.

When colour melts into your skin and when it doesn't show when you hold the mirror a foot away, that's your colour! And that colour will help even out the areas on your face that show a bit of redness or imperfection.

Now, your skin type will help you determine which formulation will work the best. As we age (yes, unfortunately, once again with the aging), our skin loses moisture, so we need a foundation that doesn't absorb any remaining moisture but retains and maybe even *adds* moisture.

And because we might have just a few more imperfections showing through than we did when we were younger, we need coverage. So find a foundation that gives you a medium to full coverage.

Tinted moisturizers may add a little colour but usually give a sheerer coverage. A matte finish is quite beautiful on mature skin. But if you want a little more luminosity, that is fine. With the new formulations, getting good coverage doesn't mean you have to have a flat looking makeup or that the application has to be heavy. If you go to a professional, then you know that you will get the right colour, formulation, coverage and finish.

## FOUNDATION APPLICATION

You can apply foundation in a variety of ways, but many of us prefer to use our fingers. If, however, your skin is oily, using a sponge or brush is a better way to apply foundation. That way, you won't get any of the oils from your fingers onto your face.

A sponge is easy to use, and it is disposable. The most common type is the wedge sponge, which can be purchased at any pharmacy or makeup store. But there are a number of makeup brands that make specialty sponges for foundation products, and they come in a variety of shapes: oval, round, even conical, that fit into the small areas of your face.

Brushes are becoming extremely popular now. There are brushes that can be used in both liquid and powder foundations.

## SKIN PRIMERS

The majority of makeup companies now have primers. Primers "ready" the face for the foundation, in the same way that a primer prepares a wall for paint (a heavy-handed explanation, but it really does work that way).

Some primers claim that they decrease the appearance of pore size and even out the skin tone before the foundation is applied. Primers aren't an absolute necessity before the foundation application, but if you find that the makeup isn't gliding on as smoothly as you'd like or you have enlarged pores, you might want to try a primer.

Today, there are bb crèmes and cc crèmes, and by the time you read this book, we might be halfway through the alphabet!

Each lotion and potion that is introduced will have very different formulations, claims, colours and coverage among the different makeup companies. Most companies will give you a sample to try. Take advantage of this offer.

Once you are fitted with your perfect foundation, your palette is ready to be painted á la *grace* style.

## CONCEALER

The eye area in particular is prone to showing age. The eye is encased in a socket surrounded by bone; this means that with aging, the eye naturally recedes. Whether it's due to genetics, lifestyle or diet, and with the skin around our eyes much more delicate to begin with, many of us see those lovely dark mauve shadows beneath our eyes, a darkness that seems to call attention to our aging.

Sigh. This is not where we want to see mauve! (And mauve, for many of us, is a gentler, nicer way of describing those deep, dark shadows we see in the mirror. However, let's be gentle with ourselves and continue to use "mauve.")

So, what can we do about it?

Concealer is a product that not only covers the darkness beneath the eye but also can be used to cover up blemishes, age spots (another lovely thing that happens as we age) and other small imperfections.

Many women *love* concealer.

Most of the time, however, I don't wear concealer. I have those eye bags, but I prefer using the *grace* method of "bait and switch." In other words, I use makeup to its best advantage by drawing attention to my best features.

In essence, this is the focus of all the information I'm giving you: *Celebrate what you love, and what you don't love will fade away.*

Because, guess what? It *works!*

However, for some women, putting on concealer is as much a part of their beauty routine as applying lipstick. If you don't want to give up using concealer, let's look at what can be done to find the best one for your skin.

First, what, exactly, is concealer?

It's simply a more heavily pigmented foundation.

Unlike television and film actors—who have the perfect lighting on them at all times—we live in real life. In real life, lighting changes all the time. This means that your under-eye concealer must not only colour that lovely mauve and the eye bags, it must look like part of your skin.

I like the simplicity and ease of using foundation under my eye during the day. This is my "concealer," and it helps even out the skin tone.

However, for special evening events? With softer light and time to properly apply concealer?

I pull out all the stops!

And concealer is one of the stops I pull out, although instead of the more traditional concealer, I use an eye brightener.

An eye brightener is a sheerer and less pigmented product that adds lightness and brightness under the eye, thus giving a brighter and more open eye.

Most of these products come with a built-in brush. You simply apply the brightener under the whole eye area and then brush it along the top of the eye bone to lighten up the area. Foundation is applied lightly on top to even out the colour.

If you use powder, simply use a clean fluffy brush to go over the area. If you use liquid makeup, apply it on top of the concealer and then fluff with a translucent powder.

If, however, you choose to use the traditional concealer, there are a myriad of choices. The most common are the small pots or wands that come in a tube.

If you are warm, use a more neutral, warm undertone concealer. If cool, choose one that is more pink-based. In your correct undertone, warm or cool, find a shade or two lighter than your foundation and skin tone.

Depending on the type of concealer you have, use either your fingers or a brush.

Starting at the corner of the eye, about an eighth to a quarter inch under the eye, apply the concealer to the entire area in a half-moon shape. Starting in the corner gives you the greatest deposit of colour there, which is where you want it, since the deepest darkest mauve is there.

Using a clean finger, gently *tap* the product into the skin. The warmth of your finger will melt the concealer. Next, apply a very thin veil of foundation over the area. If you use a liquid foundation, then use a translucent powder or setting powder over that area.

## MY *jane iredale* CHOICE

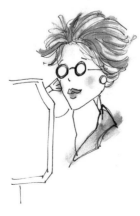

I love layering my *jane iredale* makeup for that flawless look.

*jane iredale* Glow Time Full Coverage BB Cream creates a flawless skin and is amazing on mature skin. Apply a dot of Glow Time Full Coverage BB No. 7 Cream, about the size of a pea, on your *grace* Makeup palette. I use my liquid foundation brush and drag a very small amount of Glow Time onto my brush and place it on the cheek area of my face, blending out and then using what remains on the brush around my nose and under my eyes as you would a concealer. I continue this technique until I can see an even complexion. I make sure I am feathering the foundation from the middle of my face out towards my jawline and hairline.

I then use my flat-top powder foundation brush. I press the flat-top brush into *jane iredale* PurePressed Base Mineral Foundation Powder; I look at the brush once I have loaded it with product to make sure I have used enough pressure to pick it up. I stipple, starting again on the large area of my face, and I apply what is left on the brush in the eye area. I reload the brush with the pressed powder foundation more than once.

These two products can be used alone or layered together, depending on the finish and look you want.

When I hit the gym in the morning, the H\E Dry Sunscreen NO.3 Pure Mineral Foundation—very similar to the *jane iredale* PurePressed Mineral Base formula but with men in mind— is my go-to for that one minute application before I head out the door.

However, if I am going out for a special event and want to look my amazing best, I will use my eye brightener *jane iredale* Active Light No. 4 concealer under the eye area. Unlike heavily pigmented concealers, eye brighteners add light to the under-eye area opening and giving a brightness to the eye area. *jane iredale* Active Light No. 4 is very flattering on most women with a light to medium undertone. I don't use a concealer on myself in a yellow warm undertone, as using yellow around the eye can give an unhealthy jaundiced look. The slight pink of the Active Light No. 4 is very flattering on most complexions of a light to medium tone. I use the brush included or my concealer brush under the eye, including into the corner of my eye, and bring it underneath and to the outside corner of the eye. I use my concealer brush to blend and smooth the Active Light No. 4 under my eye.

I use a small fluffy blending brush and go over the concealer with my powder foundation to blend and perfect the application.

# Chapter 5

# All About Eyes

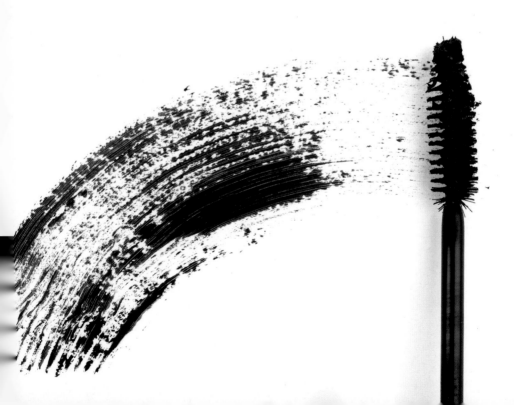

"The beauty of a woman
must be seen from in her eyes,
because that is the doorway
to her heart, the place
where love resides."

—*Audrey Hepburn*

No doubt many of us, perhaps all of us, would look at photographs of women like Audrey Hepburn and think how easy it would be "if only I were that beautiful." But it's important to notice that Audrey Hepburn connected her beauty not with her physical appearance but with what she *felt* inside.

Many things happen to our bodies as we age.

Some of the not-flattering and definitely unwanted changes can be quite easily camouflaged or covered up. A flowing fabric will skim over many a "problem" area. A peplum cut jacket enhances a no-longer 24 or 30 inch waist. Spanx will hide extra weight, while a good bra will uplift. The right clothes will help enhance our older bodies to bring out the best.

Unfortunately, we cannot hide our eyes from ourselves or from those talking to us or looking at us.

And unfortunately, the appearance of our eyes changes as we age and can change considerably. All of us will experience a more hooded eye. Aging causes a loss of collagen and elastin, as well as fat. Fat plumps up an area and gives shape and smoothness. Collagen and elastin "hold" us up, so this aging combination will show up especially in our eyes. The skin is pulled by gravity and droops (what a horrible word, but that's exactly what it does), thereby giving the eye a more hooded look.

And doesn't *that* sound simply wonderful?

No? Well, I'm definitely with you there. I'm fairly certain that none of us, not even those of us who accept aging positively, want to actually *see* the crumbling process.

So, what can we do to stop the loss of all that fat (besides wishing we'd lose it from other parts of our bodies so easily) and elastin and collagen? Is there anything we can do?

No.

It's sad to realize that elastin and collagen, youth's wonderful natural gravity-defiers, eventually become things of the past. But—and this is a big but— there is so much we can do to minimize the effects of aging, and there are ways to maximize our beauty.

Knowing your eye shape is an important first step. It will allow you to individualize your eye makeup in the *grace* way.

## EYE SHAPES

Before starting this section and talking about eyes and makeup, I just want to say that the best way to judge your desired makeup look is to simply look in the mirror once you've applied the makeup and see whether or not you like the result. Here are the common eye shapes:

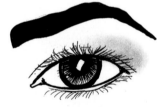

*The Classic Eye:* The eyelid is showing all the way across the top of the eye. The eyes are balanced within the width of the face. They don't tilt up or down. They are neither too deeply set nor bulging. No corrective makeup technique is needed.

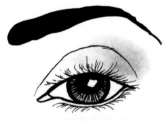

*Almond Shape/Big Eyes:* There is the "normal" balance to the eyes, but more lid and more brow shows. With this eye shape, you have a large area of lid. A thicker eyeline (using an eyeliner or pencil) will balance the eyes, where a thin eyeline won't give your eyes as much punch and drama.

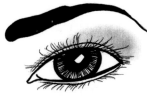

*Deep-Set/No Lid Showing:* There is no lid showing around the eye. Deep-set eyes might appear smaller, but when properly made up they are very "sexy" eyes. Use a warm or cool taupe, according to your colouring. Apply that to the whole lid area, and softly blend into and slightly above the contour. Using the contour colour this way will give the eye a sultry look, using the deep-set aspect to advantage. Keep the eyeliner close to the lashes and fine/thin, so it is more of a lash line that will define the eye.

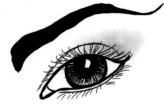

*Deep-Set/Lots of Lid and Brow Showing:* With this shape eye, you want to base the eyes from lash line to brow with your neutral base colour in the correct undertone. With the contour colour on the outside of the eye, blend upwards into the brow area and lower into the lash line, with very little into the contour. Placing a dark colour deeply into the contour will sink the eye too much. It's important to balance the eye using the eye shadow on the lower lash line. With this eye, a thicker eyeline is not only appropriate but fun.

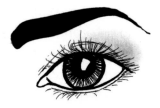

*Prominent Eyes:* The lid of the eye appears to be slightly bulging. This eye gives you a lot of lid space to work with. A thicker eyeline is necessary. Using the neutral contour taupe colour on the entire lid area, cool or warm depending on your colouring, gently blend from contour upwards into brow bone. Using the appropriate cool or warm neutral eye-base colour, place the base colour onto the brow bone area and blend into the contour you just applied so there is no demarcation line between the two colours. If you wear glasses, depending on your eyeglass prescription, this can also add to the prominence of your eye.

*Wide-Set Eyes:* The eyes appear to be set far apart. Wide-set eyes are said to be desirable. Base the eye with the correct cool or warm neutral shade. The contour colour, again the correct cool or warm for your colouring, can go a bit farther in—closer to the nose area, depending on the desired makeup look. This can be very flattering.

*Close-Set Eyes:* The eyes appear to be close together with a narrow space between them and in extreme cases can appear cross-eyed. Base the whole eye area in the correct cool or warm base colour. Keep the contour colour towards the outside of the eye to draw the eyes outward. A pop of lighter highlight colour, again cool or warm, can go in the corner tear duct area of the eye, to draw the eyes farther apart.

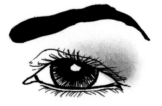

*Hooded Eyes:* Extra skin covers the natural crease, which hides the eyelid. As we get older, most eye shapes will end up with some form of hooded eye because of the loss of collagen and elastin. Base the whole eye area of lash line to brow with the correct cool or warm neutral base colour. This will take down the heaviness. Load the contour brush with the correct cool or warm colour. Place the tip in the centre of the outside half of the eye. Gently rock the brush towards the brow; this will decrease the eyebrow heaviness. Then gently rock the brush down towards the eyeline, but only about halfway. This will blend the contour line, but you want to keep the eyelid somewhat clear of contour to open the eye up.

Making your eyes more beautiful is another step to feeling and being more beautiful. But, as mentioned previously, beauty is about looking outside as well.

Find beauty in others. Take the time to really *see* the roses. Look at the infinite variety of beauty in nature. Appreciating beauty will enhance your beauty.

"I like you; your eyes are full of language."
*Anne Sexton (Letter to Anne Clarke, July 3, 1964)*

Age gives us that language, so let's add aging gracefully to our arsenal of beauty builders.

EYEBROWS

"For beautiful eyes, look for the good in others;
for beautiful lips, speak only words of kindness;
and for poise walk with the knowledge that
you are never alone."
*Audrey Hepburn*

TO MARY FROGLEY

HADST thou liv'd in days of old
O what wonders had been told
Of thy lively countenance,
And thy humid eyes that dance
In the midst of their own brightness;
In the very fane of lightness.
Over which thine eyebrows, leaning,
Picture out each lovely meaning;
In a dainty bend they lie,
Like to streaks across the sky,

Or the feathers from a crow,
Fallen on a bed of snow.
*John Keats, 1795–1821*
*(Written on or shortly before February 14th, 1816, as a*
*valentine for George Keats to send to Mary Frogley)*

"The computer can't tell you the emotional story.
It can give you the exact mathematical design, but
what's missing is the eyebrows."
*Frank Zappa*

A romantic poem and a prosaic contemporary comment written centuries apart and expressed in completely different languages each stress the importance of eyebrows. Honestly, until I was older I didn't really appreciate quite how important eyebrows are for conveying emotion and defining and enhancing the beauty of the eyes and face. More, brows underline our individuality.

Before I go on to talk about how, exactly, we go about making our brows not only beautiful but also the perfect frame for our beautiful faces, there are a couple of things we should talk about.

Many of us—myself included—plucked our brows as teenagers, to be in style, of course, because back then being in style was *everything*. And we did it without any thought to the future consequences of being so fashion forward. What self-respecting teenage girl ever thought of being over 50?

However, over 50 comes and with it the consequences of such things as over-plucking. Sad to say, those consequences can include permanent bald spots in the brows and a permanent change in brow shape.

Now adding to those consequences is an aging process that forgives no part of our bodies. While parts of our brows might have bald spots, we also have rogue hairs, ugly straight coarse hairs that sprout up not in the bald spots but everywhere else we don't want them.

Can you do anything about any of this? *Yes!*

Now, let's talk about what can be done.

The bald spots, you can colour. (See the following for details on how to do this.)

The rogue hairs, you can eliminate. Here, though, is another sad but true fact about aging that we all have to know: eventually we will have only grey and white brows. We will have brows that are not necessarily full or the shape we want, and the hairs will be coarser and longer. Then all we can do is trim the length (because length definitely isn't something we *want* in brows!), and we can fill in the gaps with dye or pencil or powder.

However, before getting to that point, colour is an option, though, unfortunately, those rogue hairs are somewhat colour resistant and therefore hard to dye. And of course, you have to make sure that the colour is right on target and the brows are dyed correctly.

Another issue: some of us have brows that somehow, mysteriously, become shorter and no longer frame the eye. Sometimes it's only one brow that is out of line because we sleep on one side. The way to handle this is with makeup. For those of you who sleep on your back and always have, you're probably lucky enough to have no pillow marks on your face and no shortened brow to worry over.

One more thing I want to discuss with regards to eyebrows: tattooing. It's a big decision, and everyone has an opinion. The *grace* opinion is, don't do it. There are of course exceptions, such as a medical condition, one that leaves no brow to work with. If, however, you have hair and a brow shape, there are proper makeup techniques that will more than likely resolve any issues.

Tattooing is permanent and will require the occasional touch-up as colour fades or changes. But if you decide it's for you, there are a few things to consider. Trying to get the perfect colour for tattooed brows can be a challenge; the colour must suit your skin undertone. For example, many women have told me that they want a natural brow or natural makeup. To that end, they look at earthy browns. But if your undertone is a cool brown, then that isn't the right colour for you. Consulting a makeup artist as well as a tattoo artist is something to explore when making your decision. Shape is also critical, perhaps more for the tattooed brow, as it can never be undone, another reason to consult both a makeup and tattoo artist.

## WAYS TO CARE FOR EYEBROWS

I present the ways to care for your eyebrows in my own order of preference. When you read this, you'll discover that you too will have a preference for which method suits you best. You might even find something that sounds better than whatever method you're using now.

- *Threading:* For me, threading is the cleanest and least traumatic to the skin. It's an East Indian method of getting rid of unwanted hair. Using a thread, the technician anchors one end of the thread and uses the other end to cut the hair. It can be a tad uncomfortable, but it is the cleanest method I have found. It is my favourite method.
- *Plucking:* Plucking by hand takes more time, but it is the least painful and something you can do yourself at home.
- *Waxing:* I find waxing is the most traumatic to the skin because pulling out the hair requires pulling on the skin. Still, there are some wonderful technicians out

there and a number of different types of waxes, so this is not a hard and fast rule.

- *Tattooing:* Tattooing is permanent. As we age, our eye shape changes, but the tattooed brow cannot be altered or changed to suit facial changes. It can fade or change colour and, if not done correctly the first time, cannot be removed. It's definitely something to think about carefully before taking the plunge.

## EYEBROW SHAPING

Whether you have one or all of the little problems associated with brows, following these *grace* steps will help you shape those brows to perfection so they frame and enhance your beautiful eyes. And your beautiful face.

There are three phases:

- *Trimming:* You need small scissors—manicure scissors work well—and a small comb, like a spoolie brush.
- *Cleaning:* Removing stray hairs around the brow area.
- *Shaping:* Tweezing hairs row by row, one at a time, to create shape.

Before beginning, clean your face of all makeup.

Pull your hair back off your face and look at your features, including your brows. (Okay, I know this isn't a favourite look for many of us, but lock yourself in your bedroom or your bathroom and consider it "me" time.)

When shaping and sculpting the brow, take all your facial features into consideration. You must look at the whole picture and create a balanced look. If you are petite with small features, your brows should reflect the delicacy of your look, not overpower everything else. If you have more prominent features (think Julia Roberts' beautiful smiling mouth and large gorgeous eyes), small skinny brows would look odd.

Now, on to the work part of the program. (It's not nearly as complicated as it seems by the length of the list, nor does it take nearly as much time as you'd think. And, once you know your brow shape, this all becomes very easy.)

- Clean your face, using a gentle toner around the eye area so it is product free.
- Define the parameters of your brow. Where it begins is more important than where the perfect arch lies. Wherever that arch is, it's perfect. It's you. Leave it alone.
- Use a white or skin-toned pencil and draw in reference points for the brow. Or use a makeup brush or any straight edge to determine where the brow should start and where it should end. Refer to the eyebrow sketch to show you the reference points.

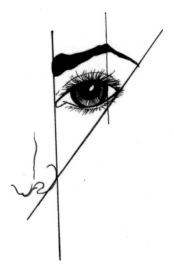

- Tweeze stray hairs first. Then work from the outside of the brow area inward. Tweeze from the root of the hair in the direction that hair grows. There will probably be some wincing. It's not entirely pain-free, but it's definitely worth it. There are two thoughts on decreasing the pain from plucking. Warming the area makes the pores open, and the hair comes out with ease. However, some women have more luck with using an ice cube to numb the area—but wrap the ice cube in a cloth so you are not putting it on the skin directly or this could cause tissue damage to that sensitive area.
- Check your work often by pulling away to gain a perspective of exactly what you're doing to make sure

you're not overdoing. Much better to under-pluck than over-pluck.

- After stray hairs are pulled, comb the brow, reassess and continue. With everything "cleaned up," move on with the shaping. Tweeze out hairs row by row, one hair at a time.
- Reassess again. Do you still have some trimming to do? If yes, comb the brow hairs up, and trim.

Now your brows are ready to be finished off with makeup!

## THE *graceful* BROW

There are a myriad of eyebrow kits, but my philosophy is simplicity. Doubling up products equals simplicity *and* efficiency. However, if you have bald spots in your brows, yet another of those unfortunate aspects that come to us all as a result of aging, I recommend using crème eyeliner because this *will* stick.

Let's begin.

First, choose the appropriate colour. If you are warm, the colour should have a warm yellow undertone. If you are cool, a cool blue undertone. I should add that 90 percent of the time, the eyeliner and eye shadow contour colour I use on someone's eye is the colour I also use on their brow. (Please see the colour section to discover your personal colouring.)

Now, choose the correct depth and intensity of your preferred colour. This depends on the colour of your brows. If your brows are white to medium brown or medium grey, you need to use a shade 25 percent *darker* in tone. For medium brown to dark grey or black brows, use a shade 25 percent *lighter*.

Next, brush the brows. Fill in any bald spots with the crème liner, then using your eye contour colour, which will be a cool or warm taupe. Using the same colour as your eye contour will bring a continuity of look and softness to the eye. Remember, this is about bringing out your best features, not about seeing the makeup on your face. It's about your look and how makeup can enhance your look and not how it can take over your look. Use this contour colour and your eyebrow brush and brush in short, sharp strokes in the direction that the hairs in the brow grow.

Use a brow comb or spoolie brush to brush the brow. This will blend the two products together to soften and give the brow that natural look.

If you find that your brows don't stay in place or that there are a few stray hairs you don't want to cut, use a brow stay product (this is a clear gel with a mascara-like wand) and brush through. Or you can spray the spoolie brush with a little hair spray and brush through.

Perfect brows!

## EYE BASE

Basing the whole eye area with a neutral colour will bring down the "heaviness" of the eye. Most women, young and old, wear sunglasses, which makes the skin around the eye appear even lighter, creating more heaviness.

While white might once have suited all of us (in our teens!), it will now make the eye appear heavier. Use a base in a neutral creamy colour with a warm (yellow) base or a cool (pink) base depending on your skin tone.

For women of colour and deeper skin tones, the powder foundation base powder you would use on your face is a better choice than an eye shadow.

This process of eye basing works well on virtually every older eye, both softening and lightening that heaviness that happens to all of us as we age.

## CONTOUR

For the eye contour, use the same colour that you use for your brow. This brings softness and continuity to your eye. Blend the correct cool or warm contour colour up to nothing, which will be about halfway between the crease and the eyebrow. This will take down any puffiness or heaviness in the brow area.

Load your brush with colour, ensuring that you remove the excess on a tissue. Place the tip of the brush in the eye crease. Go back and forth between the outside of the eye and the middle of the eye, then blend up and continue to blend out and up until no demarcation remains between the eye contour and the eye base.

See specific eye shapes for more individual instruction on shape and blending techniques.

## EYELINER

Many of us have eyeliner on our "won't leave home without it" list, and for many of us that same eyeliner was on our teen "won't leave home without it" list. But there's a difference.

As teenagers we used our eyeliner to make a statement. It was subtle or heavy, winged or smudged or smoky, but however we wore it, it worked.

For some, eyeliner is a "signature." Adele does an amazing thick and stylized eyeline that suits her fabulously big eyes and her style and makes a statement.

Unless you're trying to make a statement with your eyeliner, what is eyeliner *supposed* to do?

For the teenager, for anyone under 30 perhaps, for a star in the public eye, eyeliner is a statement, a mask, a distraction and an attraction.

But, for us "regular" gracious women? Now that none of us are under 30, we want eyeliner to shape, define, lift and pop the eye. If a thick black line is the first thing someone notices about you, the eyeliner isn't doing its job. Not that we have to stop having fun with makeup altogether, but it's best to keep the stylized dramatic look for special events and evenings.

There are many different formulations in eyeliner:

- *Cake Liner:* Uses water to activate. This creates a crisp colour-intense line. It's great for a stylized look or to glamorize an evening look.
- *Liquid Liner:* Liquid liner is intense and dense in colour. Again, it's great for that stylized evening look.
- *Pencil Liner:* The pencil is easy to use because it's soft. You can smudge easily to correct mistakes or simply to get that smoky effect. The pencil creates that soft smudged line or a thicker, more intense smudged line. The downside is that it tends to wear off more quickly.
- *Gel Liner:* These pots of gel are a little easier to use than the liquid or the cake liner as they can be more easily manipulated to create different looks or to appear smudged. The finished look is less hard-looking and stylized than the liquid or the cake.
- *Crème Liner:* With these liners you can create a softer look, rather like the look created with a pencil. However, the crème dries and stays on all day.
- *Felt Liner:* Not as common a formulation, but there are liners that are more like felt pens. They can be easier to use because you hold the felt liner as you would a pencil—which we can all do! I've found, however, that the colours are sometimes more opaque and perhaps not as deep as some prefer.
- *Eye Shadow:* A lot of women simply use eye shadow to line the eyes. This is a great alternative to other formulations because the shadow creates a soft line and it's easy to apply. A number of companies have

actually developed a clear liquid that can be added to any eye shadow to make it into an eyeliner. This works well, as eye shadow is not as heavily pigmented so the application is a little softer. Plus, a bonus is the large array of colours you can choose from. For someone with ash blonde hair and cool colouring, a grey liner creates a lovely soft look. But grey liner can be hard to find in a formulation that will create that soft look, so grey eye shadow is perfect.

There are as many different kinds of eyeliner brushes as there are eyeliner formulations. There is a small angle brush, a slightly pointed shorter brush and a long tapered eyeline brush. The best brush is the one you find easiest to use. So experiment a bit and find the one that works best for you.

## RULES OF THE EYELINE

Yes, there are rules, and my number one for eyeliner is the same as my number one rule for all makeup application: *wherever you first put your brush is where the concentration of product will go.*

My top pick for creating a defined but soft eyeline is a crème liner.

1. Load the brush with crème product.
2. Hold the brush as you would a pen or a pencil. Place your pinky finger below your eye on the cheek area to steady your hand.
3. Place the angle brush on the eyelid on the outside of the eye. Push the brush along the lash line, about three-quarters of the way across. Leave the inside of the eye, about four lashes from the tear duct, free of a line. Continuing the line right to the corner can draw

attention to those lovely mauve eye bags, which is not what you want. Also, it can close the eye, making it appear smaller.

4. If the eyeliner is not far enough along the lash line, simply begin again where you left off. It's all about practice, and I promise it will get easier to do your eyeline, and by adapting and tweaking my method you will develop your own personal application method.

5. Now, with whatever is left on the brush, place the brush on the outside of the lower lashes and again brush it along the lash line. Once again, stop short of the inside of the eye and short of that upper eyeline. The line on your upper eye should be longer.

How does an eyeline shape, define, lift and pop? Here's a simple test you can do for yourself. Create an eyeline on one eye, look in the mirror and see the pop.

1. Put on all your makeup except eyeliner. Look in the mirror.

2. Next, just do a lash line. This is where you place the eyeliner as close to your lashes as possible. This will define and pop the eye as well as making lashes appear thicker when mascara is applied. Look in the mirror again.

3. If you now make the line on the outside of your eye thicker and look in the mirror, you can see how you've reshaped and lifted your eye.

You can do the same test with the eyeline beneath the eye. You can do either a lash line to define the eye or a slightly thicker line smudged on the outside corner of the lower lash to help lift the eye.

An eyeline can help to reshape the eye by having the line thicker on the outside and lifting the eye. Some eyes can take quite a thick eyeline, as they have a large lid.

On a deep-set eye or when you want a no-liner look but want your eye really defined, a "lash line" is what you need to do. A lash line goes into the root of the lashes. This will give the illusion of thicker lashes.

Start in the same facial position as the eyeline, tip your chin and look down at your nose to open and stretch the eye. With the lash line you need to take the eyeline brush and press it into the lash line right at the lashes. There is a technique that some women use by doing little "dots" with a thin eyeline brush. The dots simply blend together, and this allows you to just press the product on the brush into the lash line area and not have to create a line and a shape with the eyeliner.

Now, once again we're back to colour.

If you are cool with ashy blonde hair and soft colouring, then use a grey eyeline for day. For evening, layering black over the grey line will create more drama.

If you are cool with dark hair and lashes, use soft black eyeliner.

If you are warm and your hair is blonde, use medium brown eyeliner.

If you are warm and your hair is deep blonde or auburn, use chocolate-brown eyeliner.

## EYELINER TATTOOING: DO OR DON'T?

I can only say one thing about tattooing on an eyeliner line: Don't.

There is a place for facial tattooing, but eyeliner is not the place to start. Eyeline styles change like any other trend, and the eyeline that suits you at 30 will not look the same at 50. For example, if you line the eye all the way in to the corner, it will age your eye and draw attention to the eye bag as you get older.

It is important to know that there is a different way of doing your makeup now, and anything you did in your younger years that is permanent will not look the same and will not bring out your best features.

Trying to cover up or alter anything permanent with simple makeup is incredibly difficult and very high maintenance.

What colour do you use? Perhaps black liner looks fabulous on you now, but chances are it will look harsh on an older you.

Even though tattooing is permanent, very often you have to get it redone as the colour can fade and doesn't look nice.

There are times when you might just want a no-makeup look, and with permanent eyeliner it looks like you didn't clean your face properly.

## LASH GROWER

The newest products out there grow your lashes. They are a great product if used to enhance and not take over your look. If used on a daily basis they work. The problem is that everyone grows lashes that are too long and look distracting.

## MASCARA

Is mascara all that it's cracked up to be? Does it make your lashes long and thick? Yes!

I don't know many women who don't wear mascara if they wear makeup at all, because, as many of us discovered when we were teens, mascara not only adds colour to lashes that—like mine—are very fair, it adds thickness and length and luster.

There is an endless variety of mascara formulations to choose from, with every conceivable brush shape and size. There are dry formulations and much wetter ones with many choices in between. There are skinny brushes, full ones and small ones.

The choice is yours. But the technique for each is the same.

First, wiggle the brush into the lashes on the outside of the eye. Draw the brush through the lashes with an upward motion, working towards the end of the eye. This opens and lifts the eye. Once again, as with the eyeliner, do not use mascara on the last four or five lashes close to the tear duct. It closes the eye and draws attention to those eye bags.

The preceding can be repeated but only when the mascara is wet enough to draw the brush through.

I find it isn't necessary to use mascara on the bottom lashes. Very often, if you do, the mascara tends to drop and run under the eye. Instead, do a lower eye line and smudge a little eye shadow on it to pop the eye.

Back to colour and choosing the right one:

If you are cool with soft colouring, use grey mascara if you can find it. If not, go with a deep cool soft black, as brown won't suit your colouring.

If you are cool with dark colouring, go with soft black.

If you warm with soft colouring, go with brown.

If you are warm with dark colouring, go with chocolate brown or brown-black.

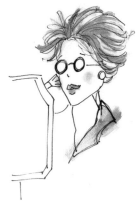

MY *jane iredale* CHOICE

The *grace* application is all about simplicity and ease of application, so in my daily makeup routine I use the following *jane iredale* colours.

*Eye Base*: My eye is slightly hooded, so I use *jane iredale* PurePressed Eye Shadow in Champagne to base my entire eye. I am quite fair, and the skin around my eye and in my eye area is very pale, so my eyes can look heavy. The minute I base my eye, the heaviness of my eye goes down.

*Eyebrows*: My next step is to fill in and shape my brows. My brows are very fair, and they don't show at all until I fill them in and give them a little colour. Also, I have some little bald spots in my brow, and *jane iredale* Jelly Jar Gel Eyeliner in brown or espresso sticks to the skin and fills those bald areas perfectly. First, I take a little *jane iredale* Jelly Jar Gel Eyeliner in brown onto my eyebrow brush (I load it, then touch a tissue to remove the excess). I gently brush the product in the brow following the natural line of the brow, filling in the areas that are needed. Then I take *jane iredale* PurePressed Eye Shadow in Cappuccino on the same brush and go over the entire brow. My final step is to use the spoolie brush to comb, soften and complete this look.

*Eye Shadow*: I prefer *jane iredale* PurePressed Eye Shadow in Cappuccino to shape and contour my eye. I load my brush and place the tip of the brush in the middle of the outside half of my eye. The tip of the brush goes into the contour eye crease with the side of the brush touching the orbital bone (eye socket) as this will allow the eye shadow to softly blend into the upper part of the eye crease. This is the trick to shape and bring the heaviness or hoodedness of the eye down. Once the brush is placed I go back and forth like a windshield wiper slowly a number of times, and then I do small circular motions towards the outside of the eye and down towards the lash line. Once the tip of brush is placed in the correct area of the eye, I do not lift the brush up and replace it anywhere else on my eye. By staying in the one place and moving the brush back and forth I create a perfect shape.

*Eyeliner*: I use *jane iredale* Jelly Jar Gel Eyeliner in brown. I load the brush and start the eyeline on the outside of my eye and create a line that is thicker on the outside and goes to nothing about three or four eyelashes from the tear duct. I use what is left on the brush to put a soft under-eye line.

*Mascara*: *jane iredale* Pure Lash Mascara in agate brown is my choice because it has a slight redness in it. This is a great colour for me as I have strawberry-blonde hair. (I never thought I would use that to describe my hair as I had bright red hair when I was younger and always thought women who had strawberry blonde weren't "real" redheads. Youth!) This colour is soft, and I like that when I use a deeper brown or even black at night it makes a big difference to my look. I don't have to use blue eye shadow to make an impact.

# Chapter 6

# Face Shaping and Blush

"The winds of grace
blow all the time.
All you need to do
is set your sails."

—*Ramakrishna*

F ace shaping is a great way to draw attention to the beauty of your face. By framing your face in the same way we frame your eyes we draw attention to the centre of your face, where the beauty lies. We can pop those beautiful cheekbones that we all love. A sweep of bronzer can also tighten up the jawline, which will also negate any demarcation line between the face and the neck.

At grace we prefer a gentler softer form of contouring. Contouring is a more dramatic way of face shaping.

Contouring is getting a huge resurgence—look at any magazine and you can see clown faces all marked up to show how you can sculpt, define and reshape your face à la Kim Kardashian. At *grace* Makeup we are definitely want to put our best face forward but with a little good taste, light hand and restraint. Clown contouring only works if you are going in front of a camera and your good friends have been lighting your shot all day. And of course you are not allowed to move, because if you do you are out of your light, and that clown contouring will certainly be showing.

Contouring is all about shading to decrease, hide or minimize a feature, and highlighting brings a beautiful feature to the forefront. At *grace* Makeup we use bronzing powders to do a little face shaping, a gentler form of contouring. By framing the face using a bronzing powder, you not only redefine your face but you add a little sun-kissed colour.

FACE SHAPES

Applying bronzer correctly begins with identifying your face shape. There are six face shapes.

Here is a list of the characteristics of each different shape. To determine which you are, pull your hair back and look straight on into the mirror. Really look at your face.

*Oval Face:* The length of your face is equal to one and a half times the width. This is the classic face shape, well balanced and proportionate. With this face shape you can wear your hair at almost any length and in almost any style.

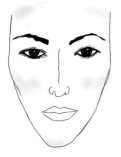

*Long Face:* You will see length in your face. You may have a high forehead or a long chin. Avoid long hair, one length, centre-part styles. These will accentuate a long face. Feathered bangs will soften the length, as will layers and a chin-length or shorter cut.

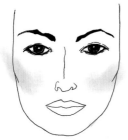

*Round Face:* This shape is fuller with a round chin and hairline, and there is often fullness in the cheek area. Keep away from short bobs and centre parts. Wispy bangs, long layering and offset parts will soften the roundness of your face.

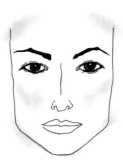

*Square Face:* This face shape has a strong squareness to the jaw and hairline. Very often a person with a square face shape has a high forehead. Hairstyles chosen should soften that squareness— wispy layers surrounding the face and forehead will help. Avoid linear cuts and very square bangs.

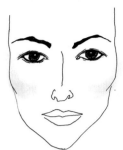

*Heart-Shaped Face*: The heart-shaped face strongly tapers towards the chin and can be slightly pointed, and as well it has wideness around the forehead. Hairstyles for this face shape should include bangs, to help narrow the forehead area and bring more fullness to the jawline.

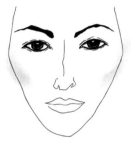

*Inverted Triangular Face*: This face shape is angular and somewhat bony and is widest at the temples. Feathered bangs and softness and layering around the jawline will help balance the face.

In the same way that you can reshape your face with the right hairstyle, you can use makeup to shape and colour your face. Using both the right hairstyle and the right makeup will give you the maximum "face shaping" effect.

Now, how, exactly, can makeup help? With shading. But it's very important that shading be done with a gentle hand so it looks soft and natural.

How is this achieved? One of the best products I've found for contouring is bronzer.

Bronzers are designed to give a natural sun-kissed colour. Just make sure the bronzer is the right shade for your colouring. Bronzers come in two or three shades. Just because you are going to use it for contouring is no reason to choose the darkest shade if you are fair.

One aside: I've seen women try to use blush to shape and contour. Blush doesn't work. You end up with badly placed blush, a too-red face and no contour. I'll touch on blush and its use later.

## BRONZING AND FACE SHAPE

In the same way that eyebrows frame your eyes, face shaping frames your face, drawing attention to its beauty. And the beauty of the face is down the centre.

Bronzer is just a fabulous way to draw attention to that beauty. But use it softly, and always brush the bronzer into the hairline, so there is no demarcation line.

Using the bronzer around the face and under the cheekbone, you will not see lines of makeup if you apply it softly. There is natural shading around the hairline, under the jawline and under the cheekbones, so you are only embellishing and strengthening the contour.

Remember when you were a teenager or in your twenties and you contoured your cheekbones and it showed? The trick today is to do it so it *doesn't* show.

When contouring under your cheekbones, first find the cheekbones. Palpate with your fingers and suck in your cheeks, and you will see the exact area to put the contour/bronzing powder. The trick as we are getting older is to start at the ear and *only contour under the cheekbone in line with the outside corner of your eye.*

Yes, it's a very small area, but if you go farther onto the face it becomes an aging line. So keep it soft and tight.

Here are some specific comments:

- *Oval Face:* Very little shaping is needed, but softly placing bronzer around the hairline will give a nice sun-kissed look, if that is desired.
- *Long Face:* If you do not have bangs, when you are shaping at the hairline, just go softly on the forehead with the bronzer to bring the forehead lower. When shaping the jawline, go a little higher on the "chin curve." Don't go too high up the chin or you will get an unnatural line.

- *Round Face*: When you are shaping your face, you want to square off the forehead and chin to give a more angled look. Cheek contour is critical here to create a more oval shape to the face.
- *Square Face*: Bronzer should be softly brushed around the hairline where the squareness is and under the jawline where there is a natural contour. You are just softening out with the bronzer.
- *Heart-Shaped Face*: Bronze/shape/contour around the hairline and the temple area. By shading the temple area, you will narrow the width where your face is widest.
- *Inverted Triangular Face*: Bronze into the hairline. Along the jawline, where the triangle face carries the heaviness, brush the bronzer slightly up the jawline and under the chin. This will narrow the lower half of your face and create a balanced shape.

This is a very simple way to create and draw the eye to the centre of the face, to the eyes and the mouth. This framing is key to a balanced makeup look, and the difference it can make is remarkable.

A note of caution if you are very fair: make sure you do not colour your hair too much going into the hairline. When your hair colouring is dark, there is a high contrast that shows in the hairline, and sometimes the whiteness of the scalp shows through, drawing the eye to that hairline. By using the bronzer *into* the hairline, the eye is drawn to the centre of the face.

## BLUSH

Blush is a very simple step that doesn't have its own chapter, but it can truly lift, brighten and finish your makeup look.

Smile and gently sweep blush on the lower part of the apple of your cheek and blend it into the contour.

Sparkles and stars and marching bands—*Voilà!* The best and perfect you!

## MY *jane iredale* CHOICE

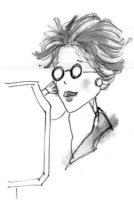

I use *jane iredale* So-Bronze Bronzing Powder 1 to shape my face and draw attention to its beauty. The face-shaping technique pops my cheekbones, tightens up my jawline, minimizes the wattle we all have, and gives me a healthy glow.

*jane iredale* So-Bronze Bronzing Powder 2 is a great bronzer I also use, as it has a little gold sparkle for the evening. The softness of the sparkle means you can use it during the day as well and the sparkle works!

For my clients who have a cool undertone, I recommend *jane iredale* So-Bronze Bronzing Powder in either 1 or 3, which has a bit of a sparkle in pink.

Blush brings that healthy glow, so smile, pop a touch of blush on the apple of your cheeks and blend back into the face contour. This sculpts and lifts your face.

*jane iredale* PurePressed Blush in Copperwind is my blush of choice as it is a beautiful soft peachy colour perfect for my skin tone. If I want a little sparkle I choose *jane iredale* PurePressed Blush in Whisper.

Sparkle is different than a full-on sheen or shine as it adds small amounts of light, and on an older face small amounts of light can be very flattering. So go ahead and put a little sparkle in your day with your bronzer and blush.

# Chapter 7

# Anatomy of Lips

"Pour yourself a drink,
put on some lipstick,
and pull yourself together."
—Elizabeth Taylor

L ips come in all shapes and sizes, and, like fingerprints, no two sets of lips are alike. Is there a perfect shape? Many think full, lush and flushed lips are perfect, but I don't think most of us have those perfect lips without a little help!

The sharp demarcation outline around the lip is called the *vermilion border*. The *cupid bow lip* is the feature where the double curve of the upper lip is said to resemble the bow of Cupid. The midline depression is called the *philtrum*.

The skin of the lips is very fine compared to the rest of the face. The lips have three to five cellular layers, and the face skin can have up to sixteen layers.

The lips contain fewer cells that produce melanin pigment, which gives skin its colour. And because there are fewer cellular layers over the lips, they look pink, as the blood vessels show through. Some people have very pink lips. The lips do not have sweat glands and do not have the protection of body oils, so lips dry out faster and become chapped more easily. Higher melanin levels offer a certain protection from UVA and UVB rays, but lips are low in melanin, and it is very important to protect them.

The lips are packed with nerve endings and are very sensitive, considered a highly erogenous zone.

LIP CARE

Drink water for beautiful lips and beautiful skin. Use lip balms with an SPF of at least 30. Use quality cosmetics. Some of the not-so-high quality cosmetics can have drying ingredients in them. Or worse!

To exfoliate your lips, take a dry facecloth and rub with a gentle circular motion. Do not use facial scrubs on your lips.

Lips can be a great indication of your true colouring. Are they more pink or mauve? If your lips are more pink, then you have a warm undertone. If your lips are more mauve, then you have a cool undertone.

## HOW TO GET YOUR PERFECT LIPS

I personally *love* lipstick. It is the finishing touch to any makeup. It doesn't matter if the lipstick is bright red or a soft flesh tone. It truly finishes a look.

There are many lip product formulations: lipsticks, glosses, balms, pencils. There are many lipstick formulations—sheers, frosted, matte and more—but most don't have the perfect applicator to really define and create the perfect lip. A lip pencil will be perfect and can create a perfect lip. Choose a colour that is as close to the lipstick colour as possible. If the colour is a little off the lipstick colour, after you have lip lined take your lip brush and blend the lipstick into the line, or you can alternately use a Q-tip.

Here are some application tips for making *your* perfect lips—a little tweaking goes a long way.

When applying lip liner, keep it touching either the inside or the outside of your natural lip line, the vermilion ledge. The exception occurs if you have what I call a *double lip line*. You can see when you look at the lip that as the vermilion line approaches the corner, there appears to be a double line. This gives you a choice of making your lips more full or less full. Isn't that great?!

When doing a lip line correction you can line the lip and fill in the whole lip with the lip pencil. However, when using a lip stain you need to apply the lip line to a clean, dry lip, so lip lining should be done after you have applied the stain. I have now developed a habit of lip lining after I apply any lipstick.

If your lips are very sharp in the cupid's bow, that can be a great stylized look, but if you want a more classic lip, gently round the cupid's bow.

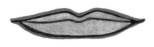

*Thin Lips*: If the upper and lower lips are thin, line the outside of the lip line. Fill the whole lip in, and no one will notice that you are making your lips fuller.

Use lighter, brighter colours. Dark colours will make your lips look finer.

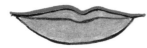

*Thin Upper Lip*: To create more symmetry, line the outside of the lip line on the top, and line the bottom lip with the lip liner on the lip line.

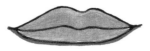

*Thin Lower Lip*: For this lip line, line the lower lip on the outside of the lip line.

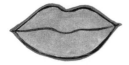

*Small Lips*: Line the whole lip with a lip lining pencil along the outside of the lip line.

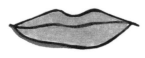

*Crooked /Uneven Lip Line*: Line the lips to create symmetry in the upper lip. In other words, if one side of your upper lip is uneven, create an even line with the pencil. No one will ever know. I worked with a television broadcaster years ago who didn't want her lips corrected even though they were "crooked," and bravo for her. She looked great.

## MY *jane iredale* CHOICE

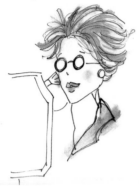

Lipstick finishes every look!

Each one of us has her favourite go-to products—and we want a lipstick that stays on. My top lipstick by *jane iredale* is Lip Fixation Lip Stain/Gloss in Craving—my go-to colour. I have tubes of it everywhere in various bags and pockets. Lip Fixation Lip Stain/Gloss is one of my top sellers, as it stays put on the lips for hours! I like a matte lipstick look, so I let the Lip Fixation Lip Stain/Gloss dry and don't add the lip moisturizer on the other end of the wand, but if you like a little moisture and shine you can use it, and the lipstick will continue to stay put. The colour "Craving" is a warm lipstick in a soft peach, which defines my lips, but it is very neutral, and I like that.

For women who have a cool undertone and want a neutral colour, *jane iredale* Lip Fixation Stain Gloss in Compulsion is gorgeous.

For a neutral colour that both warm and cool can wear, *jane iredale* Lip Fixation Stain/Gloss in Fascination is a beautiful colour. It has a slight pinky overtone and shows your lips off but is still somewhat neutral.

If you are a little more adventurous, *jane iredale* Lip Fixation Stain/Gloss comes in some bold colours as well.

My new favourite lip product is *jane iredale* PlayOn Lip Crayon. I love the colour "Yummy," as layering it on top of my *jane iredale* Lip Fixation Stain/Gloss in Craving takes the colour to a more vibrant spring tone.

# Chapter 8

# Glamour and Glitter for Evenings Out,

## Simple and Easy for Daily Life

"Simplicity is the keynote
of all true elegance."
—*Coco Channel*

For creating an elegant evening look, use a little bit of sparkle and shine. Lighting at night is softer, and glitter and shine are in order.

The number one rule of glamourizing for the evening is to always build your evening makeup on top of your day look by layering the colours. By layering, you create shape and drama. Evening shades are very often darker, and if you start with a clean face and only use your evening eye shadow colours, you will get a bruised or muddy look. Not what you want!

These tips will take your look into the evening. If you are doing a smoky, darker eye, then keep your lipstick colour soft. If you are using a softer but more iridescent or frosted eye shadow, then you can use a more dramatic lip colour. Choose the eye look you would like, smoky or sparkly; then follow the rest of the tips.

You don't have to use every tip here. Pick three, and you are still ready to go for the evening.

For *a smoky evening eye*, layer a darker eye shadow colour within your day contour colour using the bullet brush, and blend with your crease brush. Note that to create a smoky eye you need to layer your colours. I use this analogy with my clients: if you drew a circle on the wall and then coloured in the circle, you would have a black hole, but if you drew a circle within a circle within a circle, you would create depth, and that is what you want to create with the layering of eye shadows: depth, not a black hole. So layering is the key to a smoky evening eye. Using the smudge brush, use the same darker smoky eye colour and go over your lower eyeline.

For a *lighter sparkly evening eye*, use your crease brush and go over your whole contour colour with a medium-toned frosted eye shadow. Go over your lower eyeline with the same sparkly colour using the smudge brush.

Following your eye shadow, add black eyeliner on top of your soft grey or brown eyeliner. Layer black mascara on top of your brown or grey mascara. Highlight the brow bone using the highlight brush and an eye shadow in a warm candlelight colour or perhaps a beautiful opalescent colour.

## MAKEUP FOR ALL OCCASIONS: THE POWER OF THREE

When going to the gym, for a morning walk with a friend or to the morning coffee klatch, I like to look fresh and awake but not be "made up." For every woman, that look might be different, so that is why I came up with the "power of three" to create a two-minute makeup routine.

I think one of the three products for every woman should be a foundation with SPF so that in one easy step you even out your skin tone and have sun protection. I think a lot of women don't see the benefit of a foundation until they find the one that feels good on their skin or come to the *grace* studio for a lesson. Evening out your skin tone is one of the most de-aging things you can do. The clarity of the skin lets your other beautiful features shine through. I think a lot of women gave up foundation years ago because it felt like a mask, and I know I wouldn't want to feel like I was wearing a mask. So finding the right foundation will make all the difference.

The first of my power-of-three products is *jane iredale* Pressed Powder Foundation for Men 3. The other two products are *jane iredale* PurePressed Eye Shadow in Champagne, as it takes down the heaviness in my eye area, and *jane iredale* Lip Fixation Lip/Stain Gloss in Craving. I can't leave my house without lipstick.

I know a lot of women won't leave the house without eyeliner or mascara, or perhaps it's eyebrow colour. For you it might be foundation, mascara and blush, or foundation, eyeliner and mascara.

Whatever you choose, sticking with three simple products can make a big difference, and in a minute or two you are out the door feeling fresh and awake.

## MY *jane iredale* CHOICE

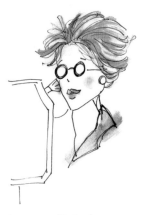

For my quick into-the-evening-look I add *jane iredale* PurePressed Eye Shadow in Steamy over my already applied day eye shadow. Steamy pink is a great colour to add some evening sparkle to the eye and can be worn on a cool or warm eye, as it will pick up the undertone of the eye shadow you are already wearing for day.

For a smoky eye look I use *jane iredale* PurePressed Eye Shadow Super Nova. It has a slightly mauve brown undertone and has a sparkle to it. I load my brush, making sure to take off excess or I will be redoing my whole under eye. I then tap and press the colour in my eye contour on top and within my *jane iredale* Eye Shadow in Cappuccino.

Add a little highlight to the brow bone and lip gloss, and I am ready for my evening outing.

# Chapter 9

# Application Review:
## Putting It All Together

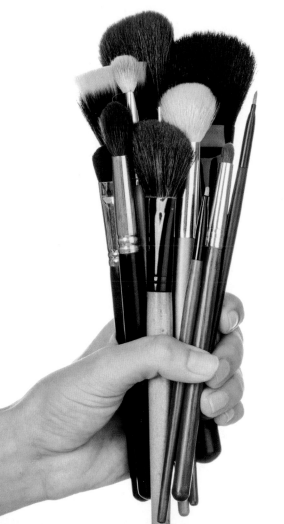

"She was a woman
who, between courses,
could be graceful with
her elbows on the table."
—Henry James

The right brushes are integral to the *grace* application. There are no hard edges on the *grace* face, because hard edges age. The key to achieving softness is to use a light hand with makeup and blend, blend, blend. It is essential. And it is flattering.

## HOW TO HOLD YOUR BRUSHES

Hold your brush exactly the same way that you hold a pen— not too far along the shaft, or you won't have complete control over the brush, and don't choke up on your brush, or you won't be able to get easy, soft stroking movements.

To load the brushes, gently place the brush in the product liquid or powder. If the brush shape is such that it has a tip to it, as in the crease eye shadow brush, don't put the tip right on the makeup product or after a while you will damage the bristles. Instead go gently back and forth with the brush on the product. It will get into the tip through this motion. When your eye shadow is running out, beware of the metal bottom of the palette, as it will damage the hairs of your brush.

After loading your brush with the makeup, work the product into the brush. If the product is liquid, go back and forth on your *grace* palette to work the product in. If you are using a powder, tap or stroke your brush gently back and forth on a Kleenex to work the powder into the hair of the brush and take off the excess so it doesn't fall on your face when applying.

Wherever you first place your brush will get the greatest deposit of colour. If using a powder foundation, eye shadow or blush, keep the brush on the face by moving the brush where you want it and not lifting and replacing the brush. This way you will have less makeup spillage on the face.

## EASY STEP-BY-STEP BRUSH APPLICATION
This is the order I apply my makeup:

1. *Primer:* Apply with the liquid foundation brush.
2. *BB Crème or Foundation Crème or Liquid:* Use the same foundation brush.
   - Start the foundation in the cheek area (the largest area).
   - Go around the nose and under the eyes. Make sure to get around the nose area and mouth area and under the eyes as you would with a concealer.
   - Reload the brush and do the forehead.
   - Tip: Always feather the product towards the outside of the face just before you need to reload. This will ensure no demarcation lines, and your makeup will look natural and not masklike.

3. *Powder Foundation:* Load the powder foundation brush and stipple onto the face.
   - Make sure you have enough product on the brush by looking at the brush.
   - Tap and press the powder onto the face. The powder will grab onto the face. This is the nature of mineral makeup.
   - You can use a smaller finishing brush if you like to get under the eyes and around the nose.

4. *Eye Base:* Use the eye base brush.
   - Load and place the brush on the eyelid from lash line to eyebrow.
   - Go back and forth gently to apply the product to the whole eye area.
   - If you use your foundation powder as an eye base, load the base brush with your foundation powder.

5. *Eyebrows:* Please see the eyebrow section in chapter 5 for details.

6. *Eye Contour and Eyeliner:* For eye contour and eyeliner, it's not always about how to hold the brush but about how to hold your face. As we get older we lose tightness in our face and particularly in our eye area.

   • To make the application of eye shadow and eyeliner easier, create tightness in the eye area by tilting the chin up and looking down at the mirror.

   • Some women apply their eyeliner by pulling the eyelid out with their fingers—ouch! I simply can't believe this is good for your skin or your wrinkles.

Here is my procedure for applying eyeliner:

• Look straight into a mirror.

• Use your index finger and push your chin up (you will now be looking down at your nose). This will stretch the eye area open and tight.

• Keep your eyes open, as it is virtually impossible to apply eyeliner to a closed eye.

• Start your eye line on the outside of the eye. The eye line should be a little thicker at the outside of the eye to lift the eye. Remember that wherever you put your brush first is where you will get the greatest deposit of colour. Do not take the eyeline right into the corner of the eye; it will close the eye and draw attention to your eye bags.

• End the eyeline softly about three or four lashes in from the corner of the eye.

• You can rest your pinky finger on your cheekbone while you are applying your eyeliner to give you extra stability and a steady hand.

To apply eye shadow,

- Look straight into the mirror. Mentally divide your eye in half vertically.
- Place the crease eye shadow brush in the middle of the outside half of the eye. This will place the brush one-quarter of the distance from the outside of the eye in the eye crease.
- Tip your chin up just a little so you see the whole eyelid area.
- Go back and forth with the brush like a windshield wiper, only going halfway towards the inside of the eye.
- Then, do small clockwise circles going downward towards your eyelashes to continue to blend the eye shadow and create a soft line. The side of the crease brush should be touching the orbital bone. By moving the brush back and forth in the crease, you blend the contour eye shadow colour just above the crease line. This is the key part of the application that reshapes the eye and softens the heaviness of the eye.
- Remember, once the brush is placed in the eye contour area, you do not move the brush to another area of the eye. Just do your windshield and circular movements down and towards the eyeline.
- If you did not get enough strength of colour in the contour, repeat the procedure.

7. *Mascara:* Apply your mascara from the root of the lash. Sweep the brush up and out towards the outside of the eyes. This will create a lift in the eye.

Make sure not to only tip the lashes with mascara as this can give a heavy look to the eye. Mascara must coat and go through all of the lashes to give a lustrous look.

8. *Bronzer:* Use your bronzer and the dome brush for face shaping, softly blending bronzer into your hairline, under your cheekbones and under your jawline and down under your chin.

9. *Blush:* Smile. Using your blush brush, put a little blush on the apple of your cheeks and sweep up and into the bronzer to create a soft and natural look.

10. *Lips:* Apply your lipstick and a little lip liner. Voilà! You are ready to go!

## MY *jane iredale* CHOICES

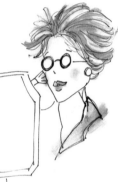

Here is a list of the products I use and the brushes, in order of application:

- *jane iredale* Smooth Affair Primer Liquid, applied with liquid foundation brush
- *jane iredale* Glow Time BB Cream in No. 7 Liquid, applied with liquid foundation brush
- *jane iredale* H\E Dry Sunscreen No. 3 Powder, applied with foundation flat-top brush
- *jane iredale* PurePressed Eye Shadow in Champagne Eye Base, applied with eye shadow powder brush
- *jane iredale* Jelly Jar Gel Eye Liner in Brown to fill in eyebrows, applied with eyebrow brush
- *jane iredale* PurePressed Eye Shadow in Cappuccino on eyebrows, applied with eyebrow brush
- *jane iredale* PurePressed Eye Shadow in Cappuccino for eye contour, applied with eye crease brush
- *jane iredale* Jelly Jar Gel Eye liner in Brown, applied with eyeline brush
- *jane iredale* PureLash Lash Extender and Conditioner
- *jane iredale* Pure Lash Mascara in Agate Brown
- *jane iredale* So-Bronze Bronzing Powder 2 for face shaping, applied with dome brush

- *jane iredale* Lip Fixation Lip/Stain Gloss in Craving
- *jane iredale* PurePressed Blush in Copperwind, applied with blush brush
- *jane iredale* Hydration D20 Spray to set and leave a dewy look

I carry *jane iredale* Hydration D20 Spray in my purse to refresh and reset my makeup for evening. And I love, love, love the fragrance!

# Warm

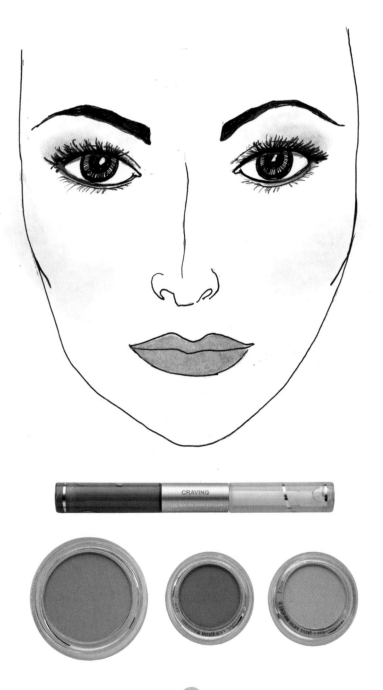

# Cool

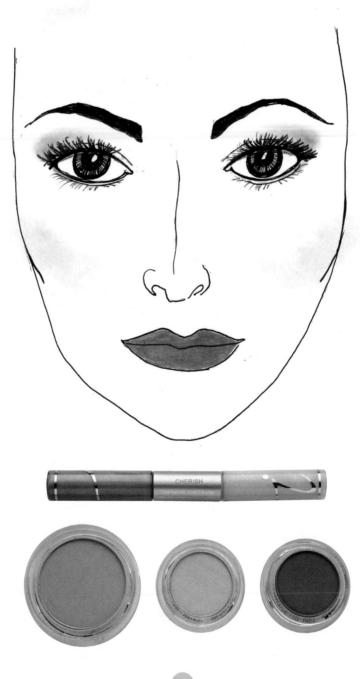

# Chapter 10

## *grace*
## Makeup
## Corner

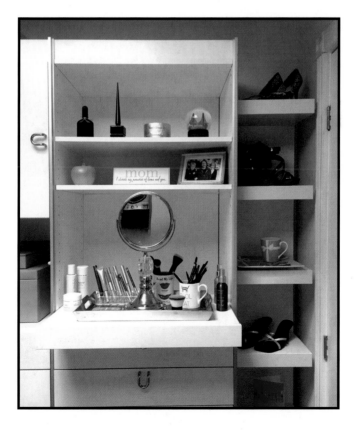

"The life I live is created
by the story I tell."
—*Abraham-Hicks*

Once you start your *grace* Makeup journey, you will want to set up your makeup corner.

In order to apply your makeup in the morning with ease and joy, you need to have an organized area. Applying your makeup is like cooking. You need the right equipment and ingredients and space to successfully bake a cake. Or to apply a beautiful face!

There's no one way or storage system, but there are a few necessities that work for everyone. I am going to touch on each of these topics so that you can set up your makeup corner and bring your own personal style to it.

For your makeup corner you need makeup, brushes, a mirror, great lighting and a space to set this all up so it's right at your fingertips—easy to access and easy to maintain. Your makeup corner should be in a ready-to-use position.

A bathroom is only a good place if you have the space to set up your products and tools without them falling into the sink. It's not a good space if it's your only bathroom and you will be interrupted at any time. I personally have a small bathroom, and only one, and I don't want to have to schedule my time in there. I prefer low lighting in my bathroom, so I set up my makeup space in another area.

I am lucky enough to have a lovely walk-in closet. It's not so big that I can set up a full vanity with a large makeup mirror and a chair just to apply my makeup, but I have a lovely space where I can designate one small corner just for my makeup. There is also a skylight in that room, which, at most times of the day, gives me some nice natural lighting. When there is not enough natural light, I can turn on the bright ceiling light.

There are a number of makeup system kits, and some cosmetic companies have cosmetic bags and kits to hold their specific makeup. I am not a big fan of these systems as they are more like jigsaw puzzles that only hold certain shapes and sizes. Makeup packaging changes and new products come out all the time, so I tend to use a more universal system so any and all shapes and sizes can fit.

## FIRST FIND YOUR SPOT

You need a minimum 2 foot by 3 foot area for your makeup corner, and if it is by a wall you can utilize the wall space. If you have a couple of drawers, that's great. If you have no wall space or drawers but have a tabletop or any similar space, there are some great storage bins on wheels that include either a number of drawers or bins similar to what hairdressers use. This is something that you can move into a corner and bring out when you need it. There are so many containers and organizing stores around, you will definitely find a storage system that will work for your makeup needs.

Makeup corners are like your purses; the bigger the bag, the more you will put in it. So if you have a large area to play with, that's great, but know that you will fill the space allotted with your makeup, lotions and potions.

## SORTING THROUGH YOUR MAKEUP COLLECTION

Gather up all your makeup, lotions, potions and makeup brushes, and dump them all out on your kitchen table. Grab some paper towels and vinegar-and-water spray to start the sorting, throwing and cleaning process. It is time to go through all your makeup and get rid of everything that is old or in the wrong colour.

I know it's hard to give up a new makeup that you just bought, but if the colour doesn't work for you, give it to a friend. She will love it! There is no point in keeping and wearing makeup that does not suit your colouring. The only person who can wear makeup in the wrong colouring is your teenage daughter.

Do a smell test. If a makeup has an odour, toss it. If a lipstick or a crème product is old it will have a bad smell or it will separate in the bottle. If you can't remember when you bought something—toss it! If you never wear it—toss it! You might have some evening makeup that you don't use very often or as often as your everyday look, and that is OK. Your evening makeup does not have to be as readily available as your everyday makeup.

A lovely woman came to me who had so much makeup, it was incredible: a huge carrying case of at least three dozen lipsticks, and more than that in eye shadows and blushes, etc. She was delighted when I told her that she did not have to change her application and makeup colours daily! It isn't *au courant* to match your makeup to your wardrobe and never will be again in our lives. I could see her physically relax.

The whole idea is to have a simple *grace* process of applying your makeup. And once you know your colouring, there is no need for more than one colour blush or a couple of eye shadows for your day look.

The only person who knows that you change your look every day is you, unless of course you are wearing a completely different colour. And if you are over 50, you don't need blue or green eye shadow!

It's about streamlining and simplicity!

Now, mentally go through every step you take in applying your makeup. Take every brush and product you use on a daily basis, and put them to the side. You should have about seven to nine brushes and anywhere from nine to twelve products. And if you are a product junkie, you probably see after this step that there are a lot of products you don't need or use daily.

If you are someone who is only just starting your makeup journey, even these nine to twelve products can seem overwhelming, but makeup application is a process.

THE SET-UP

For much of my makeup, I use clear acrylic trays that have many compartments. These clear acrylic trays work well for foundations, blushes and eyeshadows of almost any size.

The trays that hold lipsticks are pretty standard, so they are a good universal holder. I put my lipsticks, lip pencils, mascara and any other products that are in a stick form into these lipstick holders.

You will need a space for makeup sponges and Q-tips. There are a few containers that are specifically for Q-tips, but you may want to pick up a pretty container with a lid that has a lovely saying or shape or colour that will personalize your space.

I always use coffee mugs for my brushes. I use mugs that I love, love, and love! I have wonderful sayings that make me smile in the morning. It's cost effective and fun and will define your personal style.

Lighting is always tricky, as it's all about seeing what you are doing. I use full spectrum bulbs, which are touted as being as close to daylight as you can find. I do believe if your makeup looks great in the daylight it will look good in any light. Daylight shows it all! You also want to make sure your light is even on your whole face. You can't see what you are doing if half your face is in the shadow.

And you can't see what you are doing without a good mirror. At this time you might need a magnified mirror—I know I do. There are a myriad of shapes, sizes and magnifying strengths at many department stores, so you can customize the shape and size for your space. Get one with a normal magnification and one with a magnification that allows you to apply eyeliner easily.

Now for the fun part!

Put it all together. Look at your space. Find your favourite mugs, and put your clean brushes in them. Add your sponge and Q-tip container, and set your mirror up. Take your acrylic trays and put in your foundation, shadows and blush. You might have to tweak your makeup corner—enjoy the process! You will be on the lookout and find something that will be perfect for this or that. Or someone will give you a gift and the box it comes in will fit one of your products just right. You may receive a beautiful glass or mug and find that it's just too beautiful to drink out of, so you put your special brushes in it.

This is your space done with your style. Enjoy!

## YOUR ON-THE-GO KIT

I like to keep an on-the-go kit for my cosmetic and beauty products so when I go away for a weekend I just pop the kit in my weekender.

I don't double up all my products, but when my foundation or any other of my makeup products are nearing the end but still usable, I put them in my cosmetic bag for travelling. I don't want to travel with brand new products or empty my makeup drawer when I am leaving. If you don't have a separate bag, then you can't pack your makeup until you have done your makeup.

When I return I want as little stress as possible. I want my beauty regimen ready to go when I am home and ready to take with me when I am on the go. The only thing I double up on is lipstick, as I want one in my cosmetic bag and one in my purse. Lipstick is the one thing I leave the house with, and I want a spare in case I lose one.

You might want to get two cosmetic bags ready to go, one for travel and one for the gym. There are certain products that you go through faster than others, and there will always be one that is emptying out and ready for your kit.

Sample lotions and potions are great to pack for travelling, and you won't get stopped at customs for too big a bottle. Samples are the perfect size. If there are no sample sizes, there are a lot of places that sell small containers for your crème foundations and lotions and potions.

Put all liquids and crèmes in ziplock bags as well. There is nothing worse than finding your clothes wet and stained from a leaky container.

# Chapter 11

# Final Thoughts

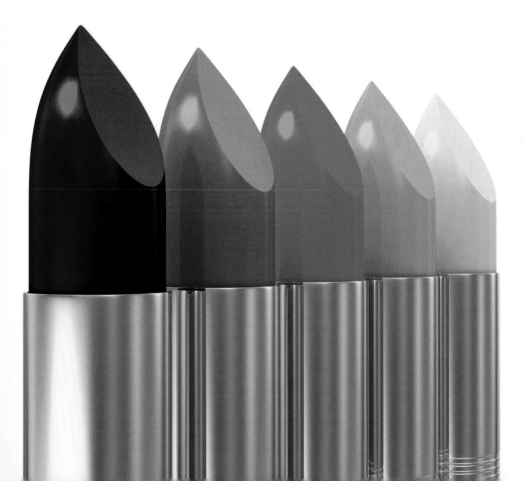

"Grace:
Simple elegance
or refinement of movement."

The word *grace* derives from the Greek word *charis*. In secular Greek, *charis* was related to *chairo*, "to rejoice." As far back as Homer it denoted "sweetness" or "attractiveness." It came to signify "favour," "goodwill" and "lovingkindness"—especially as granted by a superior to an inferior.

I never reflected on the largeness of the word *grace*. I did know that naming my company *grace* Makeup was no accident. I always knew that grace was bigger than *grace* Makeup.

Grace is about reaching out to people and being in community with your friends and anyone you are in contact with every day. I have noticed that the power of one kind word or gesture from someone is profound, and conversely, offering a kind word to someone carries equal impact.

Grace encompasses simple elegance. It really is about bringing out the beauty and elegance a woman embodies as she gets older.

It's about not being hard on yourself, about embracing what you like, loving yourself and not trying to just cover up what you don't like.

Everything that we value and love in our life has to be repeated over and over again. Everything! Because we are not perfect, and life and love and grace are not static. Every day we clothe ourselves to keep us warm, fuel our bodies with real food, exercise to keep our bodies healthy, and put on our makeup to feel our best.

The last bit of makeup I apply on clients and myself is blush. To apply blush you smile and apply.

Applying makeup is a wonderful ritual that we can practice daily. You have to look in the mirror at yourself, and this is where your day begins.

It's not about having hundreds of products to cover up or mask your face but about having the perfect key products that you double up and apply simply, easily and effectively to bring out your natural beauty and not disguise that gently used, slightly lined, slightly imperfect but beautiful face.

When I first started doing makeup, I trained with a wonderful old theatre man, Jack Medhurst. We used grease paints and our fingers. Brushes did not come till later when we had developed the right feel for makeup application. One of the most important things in my job was the knowledge that the first person an actor or host comes into contact with at the start of their day is the makeup artist, and so we as makeup artists set the tone for how that day starts.

You are that makeup artist, and you set the tone of your day. Do not apply your makeup on the train, in your car or in the badly lit bathroom of your workplace. Create a space in your home. Smile when you apply your makeup in the morning. Be kind to yourself when you apply your makeup. Make this your morning ritual.

I believe that this book will give women permission to be their best. Just by being born we have earned the right to be healthy and happy in our lives. We are meant not to fade into the shadows and hide but to rejoice in life and feel our best.

Many women I meet through *grace* Makeup have lost sight of their beauty because they are no longer "young." *grace* Makeup helps women see their beauty. I see beauty in every woman. I know that every woman who walks through my studio can feel and see her beauty when she leaves. I know that *grace* Makeup makes a difference in women's lives. It's about not putting on a mask and drawing attention to your makeup but drawing attention to your beautiful smile, the blush on your cheeks and the sparkle in your eye.

So, every day when you get up, smile as you see yourself in your mirror, brushing your teeth and moving your body. It just feels good. Make a purposeful effort every day to be kind to yourself inside and out.

It's not about perfection; it's about grace.

That is what grace is to me.

Love your age.

*Deborah Williams*